A practical handbook for
South African parents

BABY
& CHILD
HEALTH CARE

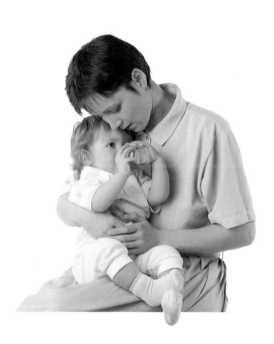

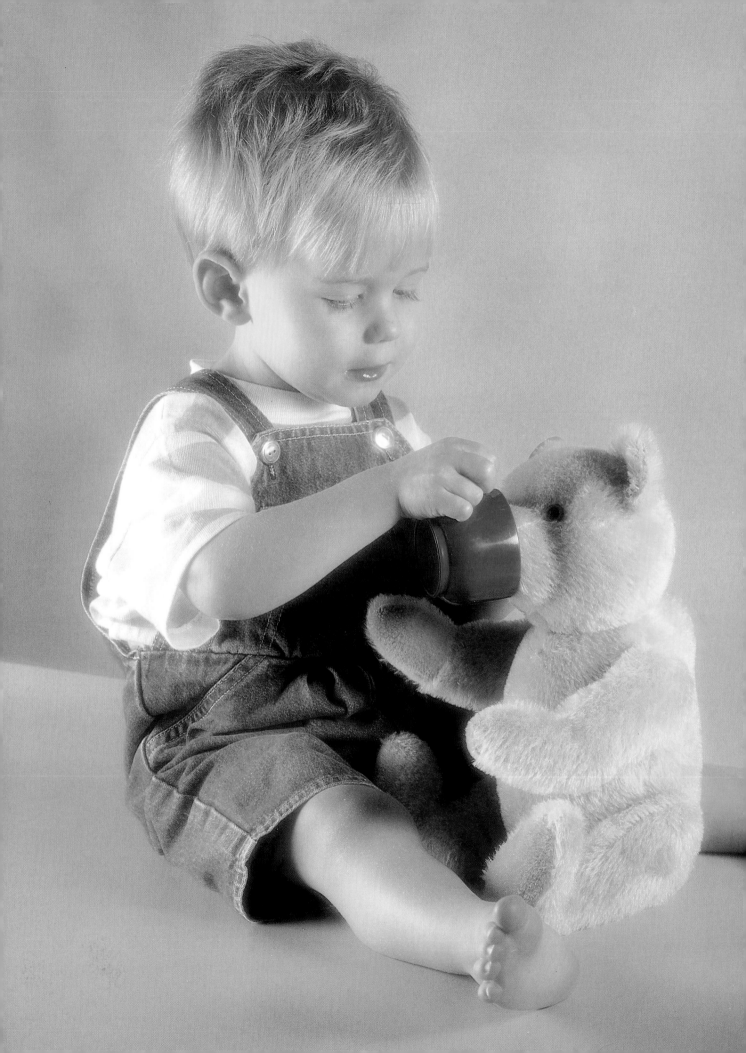

A practical handbook for
South African parents

BABY & CHILD
HEALTH CARE

Elizabeth Fenwick

STRUIK

A Dorling Kindersley Book

Senior Art Editor Carole Ash

Project Editors
Sarah Pearce, Claire le Bas;
Elizabeth Frost (South African edition)

Art Editor Tina Hill

Production Manager Michel Blake

Editorial Direction Daphne Razazan

Photographer Dave King

Consultants
Professor P. M. Leary, MD, FCP, DCH, Institute of Child
Health, Red Cross War Memorial Children's Hospital
(South African edition)
Professor Jon Scopes, MB, PhD, FRCP, Department of
Paediatrics, St Thomas's Hospital, London
Christine Williams, RGN, HV, FWT, Health Visitor and
Family Planning Nurse
Alan McLaughlin, RGN, Department of Clinical
Neurology, St Thomas's Hospital, London

First published in Great Britain in 1990 by
Dorling Kindersley Limited, 9 Henrietta Street, London WC2E 8PS

First published in South Africa in 1993 by
Struik Publishers
(a member of The Struik Publishing Group (Pty) Ltd)
Cornelis Struik House
80 McKenzie Street
Cape Town
8001

Reg. No. 63/00203/07

ISBN 1-86825-266-3

Typeset by MS Filmsetting Limited, Frome, Somerset
Reproduced by Colourscan, Singapore
Printed and bound in Singapore by Kyodo

CONTENTS

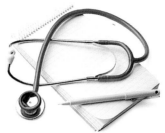

THE FIRST THREE MONTHS 6

DIAGNOSIS GUIDE 12

FIRST SIGNS OF ILLNESS 14

GOING TO HOSPITAL 17

THE CHILD WITH A TEMPERATURE 18

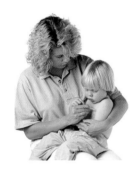

ALL ABOUT MEDICINES 21

CARING FOR A SICK CHILD 24

COLDS AND FLU 26

HAVING YOUR CHILD IMMUNIZED 28

INFECTIOUS ILLNESSES 29

EYE PROBLEMS 34

EAR PROBLEMS 36

MOUTH INFECTIONS 38

THROAT INFECTIONS 39

COUGHS AND CHEST INFECTIONS 40

STOMACH PAIN 44

CONSTIPATION, VOMITING
AND DIARRHOEA 45

BLADDER, KIDNEY AND GENITAL
PROBLEMS 48

SKIN PROBLEMS 50

EPILEPSY AND MENINGITIS 57

YOUR CHILD'S SAFETY 58

FIRST AID 61

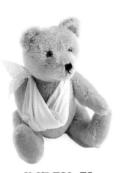

INDEX 78

ACKNOWLEDGMENTS 80

THE FIRST THREE MONTHS

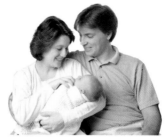

It is always difficult to know whether a baby is ill, especially with your first baby. If he seems contented, and is taking his feeds normally, he is probably perfectly healthy. But babies can become ill quite quickly and any infection may be dangerous, so for the first three months you should take no chances: be overcautious and call your doctor straight away if you think your baby is ill. If you notice any signs of illness, look at the symptoms listed below and opposite. These are the main health risks and the most common minor problems for babies under three months old. This symptom guide directs you to the relevant section on pages 8–11, but is not intended as a definite medical diagnosis – only a doctor can give that. If you can't find your baby's symptoms here, look at the guide on pages 12–13, which covers illnesses for babies and children of all ages.

Babies are born with a natural immunity to many infections, since antibodies (which destroy germs) are passed to them from their mother's blood. Breast-fed babies also receive antibodies from their mother's milk. This immunity lasts for about six months, so before this age your baby is very unlikely to catch any of the infectious illnesses that are common in childhood.

■ EMERGENCY SIGNS ■

Call for emergency help immediately if your baby:
- ▲ brings up green vomit
- ▲ has a temperature over 39°C (102.2°F) for more than half an hour
- ▲ vomits AND cries uncontrollably as if in great pain
- ▲ is breathing very noisily or rapidly

Fontanelle

- ▲ has a taut, bulging fontanelle when he isn't crying
- ▲ screams with pain and turns pale when he screams
- ▲ passes stools containing blood and mucus, which resemble red-currant jelly.

■ CALL THE DOCTOR ■

Don't wait to call your doctor now if your baby seems unwell or:
- ▲ cries more than usual, or his crying sounds different from usual over a period of about an hour
- ▲ seems abnormally quiet, drowsy or listless
- ▲ refuses two successive feeds, or does not demand a feed for six hours
- ▲ seems particularly irritable or restless.

Crying
If none of your usual soothing methods calms your baby after an hour or so, or if his crying sounds unusual, **call your doctor now**. If your baby cries inconsolably for two or three hours at about the same time each day, but shows no other signs of illness, he might have colic. This may continue for several weeks, but there is no treatment for it.

PREMATURE BABIES
Babies who were very small at birth, or who were born a month or more before their due date, are very vulnerable to infections during their first weeks. Until your baby is older and has put on weight, keep him away from anyone who has a cough or cold, and don't take him into public places where he might pick up an infection.

Cold hands and feet, *see Chilling (page 10)*

Areas of dry, flaking skin *mean that your baby's skin needs moisturizing, so rub a little baby oil or baby moisturizer gently into the dry areas.*

Loss of appetite
If your baby does not want to feed, but seems generally well and contented, there is no need to worry. If he refuses two feeds in succession, or does not demand a feed for six hours, **call your doctor now**.

Slow weight gain
If your baby does not seem to be gaining weight at the normal rate (refer to a weight chart) consult your doctor or clinic sister. Occasionally an underlying illness can make a baby grow more slowly than normal.

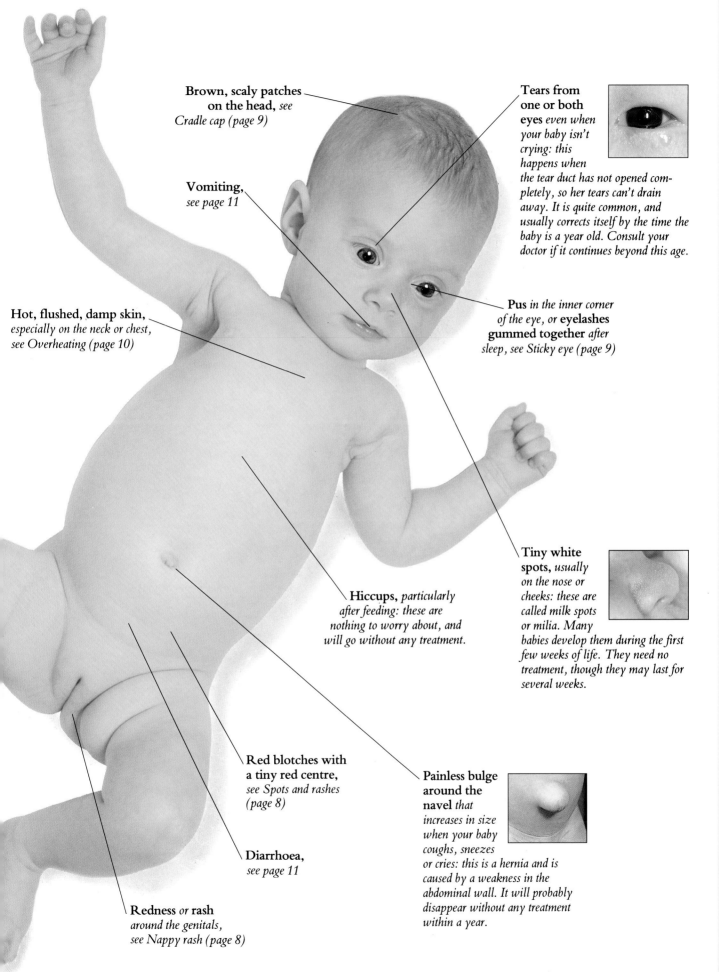

Brown, scaly patches on the head, *see* Cradle cap (page 9)

Tears from one or both eyes *even when your baby isn't crying: this happens when the tear duct has not opened completely, so her tears can't drain away. It is quite common, and usually corrects itself by the time the baby is a year old. Consult your doctor if it continues beyond this age.*

Vomiting, *see page 11*

Hot, flushed, damp skin, *especially on the neck or chest, see Overheating (page 10)*

Pus *in the inner corner of the eye, or* eyelashes gummed together *after sleep, see Sticky eye (page 9)*

Hiccups, *particularly after feeding: these are nothing to worry about, and will go without any treatment.*

Tiny white spots, *usually on the nose or cheeks: these are called milk spots or milia. Many babies develop them during the first few weeks of life. They need no treatment, though they may last for several weeks.*

Red blotches with a tiny red centre, *see Spots and rashes (page 8)*

Painless bulge around the navel *that increases in size when your baby coughs, sneezes or cries: this is a hernia and is caused by a weakness in the abdominal wall. It will probably disappear without any treatment within a year.*

Diarrhoea, *see page 11*

Redness *or* rash *around the genitals, see Nappy rash (page 8)*

SPOTS AND RASHES

What are they?

Many newborn babies go through a spotty stage, so don't worry if your baby develops a few spots – they don't mean that he is ill. One of the most common rashes is called newborn urticaria; it usually appears during the first week of life, and disappears without treatment.

What can I do?

If your baby has newborn urticaria (see symptoms box), simply ignore the spots – they will disappear on their own within about two or three days, so don't put any lotions or creams on them. Don't alter your baby's feeds – the spots are not due to milk disagreeing with him.

SYMPTOMS

▲ Red blotches with a tiny red centre, which come and go on different parts of the baby's body, and last only a few hours.

CALL THE DOCTOR

Call your doctor now if the spots are flat and dark red or purplish (a petechial rash). Consult your doctor as soon as possible if:
▲ a spot has developed a pus-filled centre
▲ you think a spot has become infected.

NAPPY RASH

What is it?

Nappy rash is an inflammation of the skin on a baby's bottom. It may occur if your baby has been left in a dirty nappy for too long, because as his urine and faeces are broken down, ammonia is released, which burns and irritates his skin. It can also be due to an allergy to soap powder or fabric conditioner used when washing fabric nappies. A similar-looking rash may be caused by thrush, which normally starts in the mouth (see page 38), but can spread through the body and affect the skin around the anus.

SYMPTOMS

▲ Red, spotty, sore-looking skin in the nappy area
▲ smell of ammonia from your baby's nappy.

What can I do?

1 Buy a nappy rash cream (available at most pharmacies) and apply it when you change her nappy, to soothe and heal the skin.

2 Change your baby's nappy frequently, and clean and dry her bottom thoroughly at each change. Inside fabric nappies, use an extra-absorbent type of liner.

3 Whenever possible, let your baby lie on a nappy with her bottom exposed to the air. Don't use plastic pants over fabric nappies until the rash subsides, since these prevent air circulating to her bottom.

Spread the cream *evenly all over your baby's nappy area*

4 Don't use biological powder or fabric conditioner to wash her nappies, as they can trigger an allergy. Rinse her nappies thoroughly.

5 Look for white patches inside your baby's mouth. If you see any, she may have thrush (see page 38).

CALL THE DOCTOR

Consult your doctor as soon as possible if:
▲ the rash lasts longer than two days
▲ you think your baby has thrush.

What might the doctor do?

The doctor may prescribe an antibiotic cream if the rash has become infected, or an anti-fungal cream if your baby has thrush.

CRADLE CAP

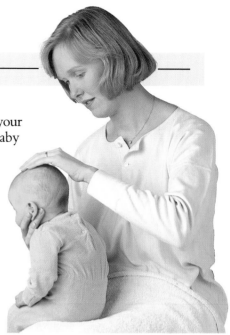

What is it?
Brown, crusty patches on a baby's head are known as cradle cap. Sometimes it may spread to the baby's face, body, or nappy area, producing a red scaly rash. Although it looks irritating and unsightly, cradle cap doesn't seem to distress the baby.

SYMPTOMS

▲ Brown, scaly patches on the scalp.

CALL THE DOCTOR

Consult your doctor as soon as possible if the rash spreads and:
▲ seems to irritate the baby
▲ looks infected or begins to ooze
▲ does not clear up after five days.

What can I do?
1 Rub the scales on your baby's head with baby oil to soften them. Leave the oil on for 12 to 24 hours, then comb his hair gently to loosen the scales. Finally, wash his hair – most of the scales should simply wash away.

2 If the rash spreads, keep the affected areas clean and dry. Don't use soap, baby lotion or baby bath liquid – ask your pharmacist for an emulsifying ointment instead.

What might the doctor do?
If the condition proves obstinate, or if the rash looks infected or starts to ooze, your doctor may prescribe a cream to be rubbed gently on the area.

STICKY EYE

What is it?
This is a very common mild eye infection caused by blood or fluid getting into your baby's eye during birth. If your baby develops any of these symptoms after she is two days old, she probably has conjunctivitis (see page 34).

SYMPTOMS

▲ Eyelashes gummed together after sleep
▲ pus in the inner corner of the eye.

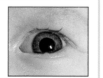

CALL THE DOCTOR

Call your doctor now if your baby has a bad discharge of yellow pus. Consult your doctor as soon as possible if:
▲ your baby develops symptoms of sticky eye after the first two days of life
▲ sticky eye does not clear up after three days.

What can I do?
Clean your baby's eyes twice a day with cotton wool dipped in warm boiled water. Wipe outwards from the inner corner of her eye, and use a fresh piece of cotton wool for each eye.

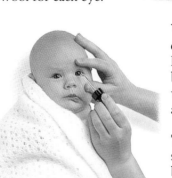

What might the doctor do?
If the doctor thinks your baby has conjunctivitis, he will probably prescribe antibiotic eye drops.

To give the eye drops, swaddle your baby in a blanket and hold her eyes open very gently, then squeeze in the drops. If necessary, ask another adult to hold her head still.

CHILLING

Why are babies at risk?
For the first few weeks, your baby cannot regulate his body temperature very efficiently. If he gets cold, his body temperature will drop and he may become dangerously chilled quite quickly. Premature babies are particularly vulnerable to this.

What can I do?

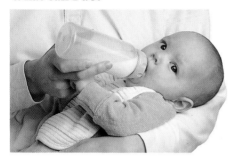

1 Warm your baby up by taking him into a heated room and feeding him. Once he has become chilled, it doesn't help just to pile on extra clothes or blankets.

2 Take your baby's temperature (see page 19). If it is below 35°C (95°F), he is dangerously chilled, so **call your doctor now**.

SYMPTOMS

First signs
▲ Crying and restless behaviour
▲ cold hands and feet.

Signs of serious chilling
▲ Quiet, listless behaviour as the baby gets colder
▲ cool skin on the chest and stomach
▲ pink, flushed face, hands and feet.

How can I prevent chilling?
Keep the room your baby sleeps in at about 20°C (68°F). When you undress and bathe him, the room should be warmer still. Be sensible about taking him out in cold weather – wrap him up well and don't stay out for too long. Never leave him to sleep outside in his pram on a cold day.

CALL THE DOCTOR
Call your doctor now if your baby:
▲ shows signs of serious chilling
▲ has a temperature below 35°C (95°F).

Put a bonnet *under the hood to keep his head warm*

In cold weather, dress your baby in an all-in-one outdoor suit, or wrap a shawl over his other clothes and use mittens and bootees.

OVERHEATING

Why are babies at risk?
Babies must be kept warm but overheating can be dangerous and could be associated with cot death.

What can I do?
1 Take your baby to a cooler place and remove a layer of clothing.

2 Take her temperature (see page 19) and, if it is raised, reduce it by tepid sponging (see page 20). Allow an electric fan to blow gently on her.

3 Dress your baby in light clothes when she seems comfortable.

SYMPTOMS
▲ Restless behaviour
▲ hot, sweaty skin
▲ raised temperature.

How can I prevent overheating?
Dress your baby according to the weather – on very hot days, she can sleep in just a nappy and a vest, but always remember the danger of chilling (see above). Never leave her to sleep in the sun, her skin will burn easily. Provide shade of some sort, and check her frequently as the sun moves round.

CALL THE DOCTOR
Call your doctor now if your baby has a temperature over 38°C (100.4°F).

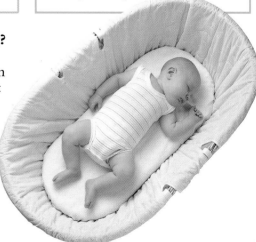

VOMITING

Why do babies vomit?
All babies bring up a small amount of milk during or just after a feed. This is perfectly normal, and does not mean that your baby is ill, but until you are used to it, you may think that she is vomiting. If your baby vomits, she will bring up most of her feed. This is unlikely in a breast-fed baby.

Frequent vomiting in a bottle-fed baby, especially if she also has diarrhoea, may be caused by gastro-enteritis (see page 46). This is very serious because it can make her dehydrated very quickly.

FORCEFUL VOMITING
Sometimes a baby vomits with great force, so that the vomit shoots across the room. If your baby does this at two successive feeds, **consult your doctor as soon as possible.**

Much the most likely reason is that she has brought back part of her feed with a large burp of wind behind it. However, if it happens after every feed, especially if your baby seems hungry all the time, she may have a condition called pyloric stenosis, in which the outlet from the stomach becomes blocked. This condition runs in families, and usually develops when the baby is about two to eight weeks old. If your baby has this, she will need a simple operation.

What can I do?

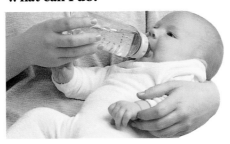

1 Stop bottle-feeding for 24 hours. Give your baby frequent drinks (30–60 ml every one to two hours) of a sugar/salt solution (half a level teaspoon of salt and eight level teaspoons of sugar in a litre of water), or ask your pharmacist for oral rehydration powder; she needs at least ½ litre (1 pint) a day.

2 Resume normal feeds once your baby has stopped vomiting and is keeping the solution in. This could take as long as 24 hours. In the past doctors advised the reintro-duction of milk feeds in a diluted form, increasing strength over several days. Research has shown that this is not necessary and, indeed, can harm the baby. Thus, once vomiting has stopped, give milk feeds of normal strength.

■ EMERGENCY SIGNS ■
Call for emergency help immediately if your baby:
▲ vomits all feeds in an eight-hour period
▲ has a dry mouth
▲ has sunken eyes
▲ has a sunken fontanelle
▲ has a dry nappy for more than six hours.

■ CALL THE DOCTOR ■
Call your doctor now if:
▲ your baby vomits and shows any other signs of illness
▲ your baby vomits the whole of two successive feeds.

What might the doctor do?
The doctor may prescribe a powder to be mixed with water for your baby to drink. If your baby has lost a lot of body fluid, the doctor might send her to hospital, where she may be given liquid through a drip.

How can I prevent an upset stomach?
Breast-fed babies rarely have upset stomachs. If you are bottle-feeding your baby, sterilize all feeding equip-ment and throw away any unfinished feeds. When you make up feeds, cool them quickly under cold running water and store in the fridge. Never keep a feed warm for a long period.

DIARRHOEA

What is it?
Until babies start eating solid food, they usually pass fairly runny stools a few times a day. If your baby passes very watery, greenish stools more often than usual, he has diarrhoea. This is serious in a young baby, since it may dehydrate him quickly.

What can I do?
To prevent dehydration, give your baby frequent drinks (30-60 ml every one to two hours) of a solution containing half a level teaspoon of salt and eight level teaspoons of sugar in a litre of water. Stop breast-feeding if your baby is also vomiting.

■ CALL THE DOCTOR ■
Call for emergency help immediately if your baby has any of the emergency signs listed for vomit-ing. Call the doctor now if your baby has diarrhoea for six hours.

DIAGNOSIS GUIDE

If your child seems unwell, try to identify her symptoms in the guide below. If she has more than one symptom, look up the one which seems to be the most severe. This gives you a possible diagnosis and refers you to a section covering the complaint that your child might be suffering from. As well as giving a more detailed list of symptoms for the complaint, the section contains a brief explanation of the nature of the illness, with information about how you can help your child, and advice on whether you need to call a doctor. Bear in mind that the guide below is not intended to give an accurate diagnosis – only a doctor can do that – and that your child may not develop all the symptoms listed for an illness. If your baby is under three months old, look also at the guide on pages 6–7, which covers special health risks for young babies.

Raised temperature
A raised temperature (fever) may mean that your child has an infection, so you should check for other signs of illness. However, healthy children may get a slight fever during energetic play or in very hot weather, so check your child's temperature again after she has rested for about half an hour. If it is still over 38°C (100.4°F), she may have an infection.

Changed behaviour
If your child is less lively than usual, more irritable, whiny or simply miserable, she may be ill.

Unusual paleness
If your child looks much paler than usual, she may be ill.

Hot, flushed face
This may be a sign of a fever.

Loss of appetite
Although a child's appetite varies from meal to meal, a sudden loss of appetite may be a sign of illness. If your baby is under six months old and has refused two successive feeds, or has not demanded a feed for more than eight hours, **call your doctor now**. If your child goes off her food for more than 24 hours, look for other signs of illness (see page 15).

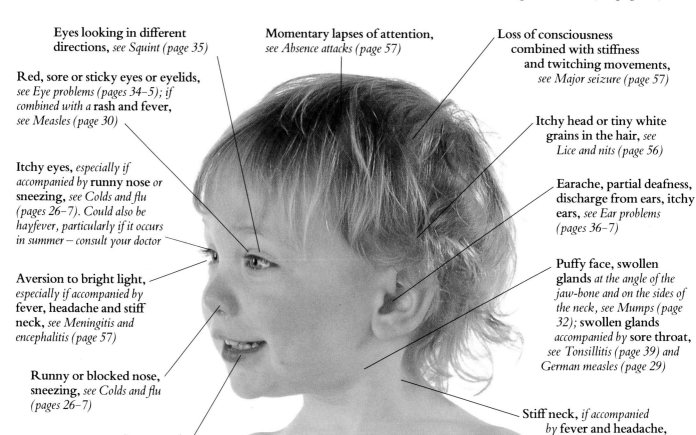

Eyes looking in different directions, *see* Squint *(page 35)*

Red, sore or sticky eyes or eyelids, *see* Eye problems *(pages 34–5); if combined with a* rash and fever, *see* Measles *(page 30)*

Itchy eyes, *especially if accompanied by* runny nose *or* sneezing, *see* Colds and flu *(pages 26–7). Could also be hayfever, particularly if it occurs in summer – consult your doctor*

Aversion to bright light, *especially if accompanied by* fever, headache and stiff neck, *see* Meningitis and encephalitis *(page 57)*

Runny or blocked nose, sneezing, *see* Colds and flu *(pages 26–7)*

Sore mouth, *see page 38*

Momentary lapses of attention, *see* Absence attacks *(page 57)*

Loss of consciousness combined with stiffness and twitching movements, *see* Major seizure *(page 57)*

Itchy head or tiny white grains in the hair, *see* Lice and nits *(page 56)*

Earache, partial deafness, discharge from ears, itchy ears, *see* Ear problems *(pages 36–7)*

Puffy face, swollen glands *at the angle of the jaw-bone and on the sides of the neck, see* Mumps *(page 32);* swollen glands *accompanied by* sore throat, *see* Tonsillitis *(page 39) and* German measles *(page 29)*

Stiff neck, *if accompanied by* fever and headache, *see* Meningitis and encephalitis *(page 57)*

Red lump, perhaps with pus-filled centre *anywhere on the body, see Spots and boils (page 50)*

Red, raw skin, *see Chapped skin (page 53)*

Sore throat, *see Throat infections (page 39); if accompanied by* fever and general illness, *see Colds and flu (pages 26–7); if also accompanied by a* rash, *see German measles (page 29); if accompanied by* puffy face, *see Mumps (page 32)*

Spots or rash *anywhere on the body, if accompanied by* sore throat *or* fever, *see Infectious illnesses (pages 29–31); if without other symptoms, see Skin disorders (pages 50–5) and Insect stings (page 76)*

Stomach pain, *see page 44; if accompanied by nausea, vomiting or diarrhoea, see Gastro-enteritis (page 46)*

Abnormal-looking faeces, *see page 47*

Diarrhoea, *see page 47*

Constipation, *see page 45*

Intense itching around the anus, *see Threadworms (page 56)*

Pain when urinating, odd-coloured urine, frequent urination, *see Urinary system infections (page 48)*

Sore tip of penis, *see Genital problems in boys (page 49)*

Painless bulge in the groin or scrotum, *see Genital problems in boys (page 49)*

Vomiting with great force *in babies, see Forceful vomiting (page 11)*

Vomiting or nausea, *see page 46*

Sores around the mouth, *see Cold sores (page 54) and Impetigo (page 55)*

Faint red rash over the face or in skin creases, *see Heat rash (page 51)*

Cough, *see Coughs and chest infections (pages 40–3) and Whooping cough (page 33); if accompanied by a rash, see Measles (page 30)*

Breathing difficulty, wheezing, rapid breathing, *see Chest infections (pages 40–3)*

Areas of very itchy, dry, red, scaly skin *anywhere on the body, see Eczema (page 52)*

Red, tender skin *anywhere on the body, see Sunburn (page 53) or Burns and scalds (page 69)*

Dry, painless lump *anywhere on the body, see Warts (page 54)*

Soreness, itching or redness around the vagina, vaginal discharge, *see Genital problems in girls (page 49)*

Intense itching around the vagina, *see Threadworms (page 56)*

White or brown lump on the sole of the foot, *see Plantar warts (page 54)*

FIRST SIGNS OF ILLNESS

Even if your child has no definite symptoms, you will probably know when he is sickening for something. You may notice that he looks pale and is more clingy than usual. He may be off his food; he may cry or whine, or seem very irritable. When your baby is teething, don't assume that any symptoms he has are due to this. Although teething may make his gums sore, so that he is more dribbly and irritable than usual, it won't give him a temperature or make him ill. If you think that your child might be ill, check for any definite symptoms, as described opposite. In a baby under a year old, all symptoms should be taken seriously – babies can become ill very quickly. If your child is over a year old, keep a check on how his symptoms progress over the next few hours.

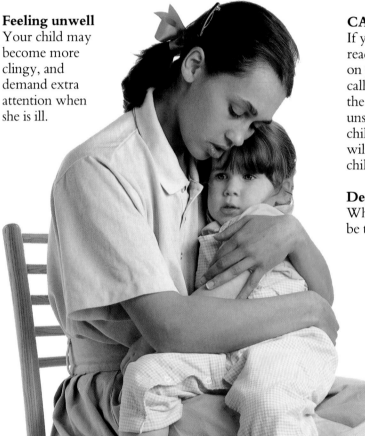

Feeling unwell
Your child may become more clingy, and demand extra attention when she is ill.

CALLING THE DOCTOR

If you think you know what is wrong with your child, read the relevant section among the complaints covered on pages 26–57. This advises you whether you need to call the doctor. As a general rule, the younger the child, the more quickly he should be seen by a doctor. If you are unsure what to do, phone your doctor and describe your child's symptoms to him and tell him his age. The doctor will tell you what to do and will know whether your child needs medical attention.

Degree of urgency
Whenever you are instructed to call the doctor, you will be told how quickly your child needs medical help.

■ **Call for emergency help immediately:** this is a life-threatening emergency, so call for an ambulance, or go to the nearest hospital emergency department.

■ **Call your doctor now:** your child needs medical help now, so contact your doctor straight away, even if it is the middle of the night. If he can't come now, call for emergency help immediately.

■ **Consult your doctor as soon as possible:** your child needs to be seen by a doctor within the next 24 hours.

■ **Consult your doctor:** your child should be seen by a doctor within the next few days.

SYMPTOMS

The most common early symptoms of illness in children are:
▲ raised temperature – 38°C (100.4°F) or more
▲ crying and irritability
▲ vomiting or diarrhoea
▲ refusal to eat or drink
▲ sore or red throat
▲ rash
▲ swollen glands in the neck or behind the jaw.

EMERGENCY SIGNS

Call for emergency help immediately if your child:
▲ is breathing very noisily, rapidly or with difficulty
▲ has a convulsion
▲ loses consciousness after a fall
▲ is in severe, persistent pain
▲ has a fever and is unusually irritable or drowsy
▲ has a rash of flat dark red or purplish blood-spots (petechial rash).

CHECKING FOR SYMPTOMS

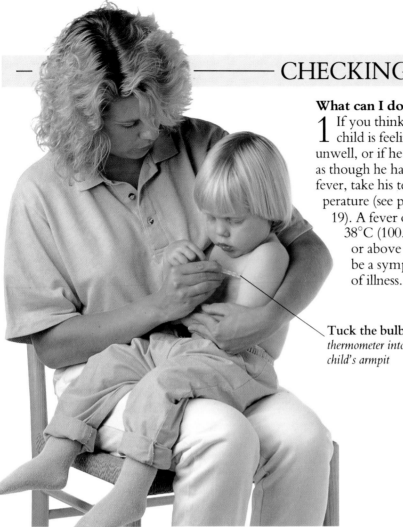

What can I do?

1 If you think your child is feeling unwell, or if he looks as though he has a fever, take his temperature (see page 19). A fever of 38°C (100.4°F) or above can be a symptom of illness.

Tuck the bulb *of the thermometer into your child's armpit*

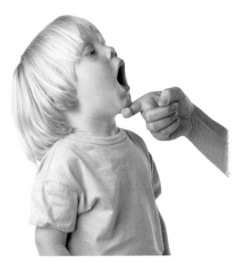

2 Check whether your child's throat is inflamed or infected, but don't try to examine the throat of a baby under a year old. Ask your child to face a strong light and open his mouth. If he is old enough to understand, ask him to say 'Aah' to open the back of his throat. If his throat looks red or you can see creamy spots, he has a sore throat (see Throat infections, page 39).

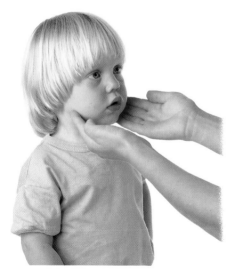

3 Feel gently along your child's jaw-bone and down either side of the back of his neck. If you can feel tiny lumps under the skin, or if any of these areas seem swollen or tender, your child has swollen glands, which is a common sign of illness.

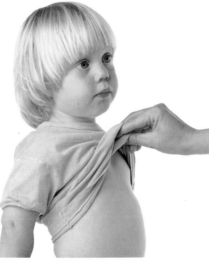

4 Check to see whether your child has a rash, particularly on his chest and behind his ears – the most common areas for a rash to start. If he has a rash and a fever, he may have one of the common childhood infectious illnesses (see pages 29–31).

QUESTION & ANSWER

"Is my child in pain?"

If your baby is in pain, his crying may sound different from normal. When a baby or small child cries or complains of pain, it can be difficult to discover where the pain is, let alone how bad it is.

Serious pain will affect your child's behaviour, so watch him to find out how severe his pain is. Does it make him cry or stop him sleeping, eating or playing? Does his face look drawn or his colour change? Would you know he had a pain even if he didn't tell you? If not, his pain is not severe.

Except for earache (see pages 36–7), don't give any pain-killers without your doctor's advice: pain helps diagnosis.

THE DOCTOR'S EXAMINATION

The doctor will ask you about any symptoms you have noticed in your child and how long he has had them, and will then examine your child. If your child is old enough to understand, explain what will happen when he visits the doctor. If the doctor suspects any particular illness, he may do other investigations as well as or instead of those shown below.

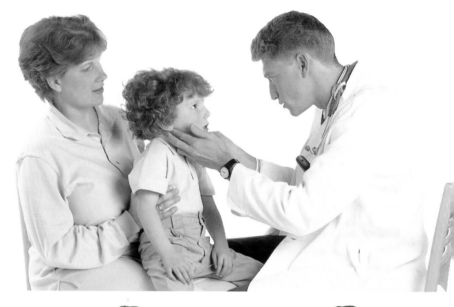

1 The doctor will feel the glands that lie along your child's jaw-bone, down the back of his neck, and in his armpits and groin. These may become swollen during an infectious illness.

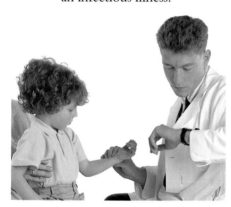

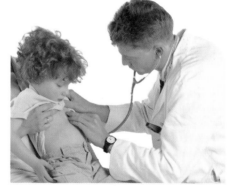

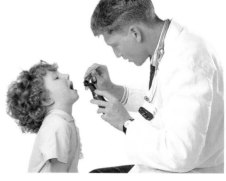

2 He will feel your child's pulse to check if his heart is beating faster than usual. This is often a sign of a raised temperature. The doctor may also take your child's temperature.

3 By listening to your child's chest and back through a stethoscope, and asking your child to breathe deeply, the doctor will check the health of his heart and lungs.

4 If your child has a sore or inflamed throat, the doctor will examine his throat using a small torch, pressing his tongue down with a spatula.

5 The doctor may ask your child to lie on the examining couch, so that he can gently feel his abdomen. He will check for swelling or tenderness in any of the internal organs.

QUESTIONS TO ASK THE DOCTOR

Don't hesitate to ask the doctor about anything that is worrying you. In particular, find out:
■ how long your child may be ill, and what symptoms to expect
■ whether he is infectious, and whether you should isolate him, particularly from small babies and pregnant women
■ how you can make your child more comfortable while he is ill.

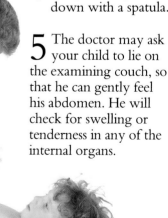

GOING TO HOSPITAL

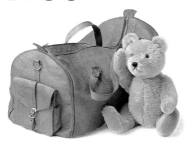

Going into hospital is stressful for anyone. For a child who is too young to understand why he is there or, indeed, whether he will ever come out, it can be terrifying, especially if it also means that he is separated from his parents. While it helps to explain to your child what is happening, you can't do much to prepare him if he is under two – all he really needs at this age is your presence. If your child is over two, playing with a favourite toy may help: explain that teddy goes to hospital to have something put right, not as a punishment, mummy stays with him or visits him as much as she can, and soon teddy comes home again. Keep your explanations simple but truthful; your child will feel let-down and mistrustful if you promise something won't hurt, and then it does.

VISITING YOUR CHILD

Hospital staff know how important it is for a parent to be with a child to comfort and reassure him, and should make it easy for you to visit him at any time. Some even provide accommodation so that you can live in with your child – find out about this before his admission. He won't find hospital so frightening if you continue to care for him as you would at home, so ask the nurses whether you can still bathe and feed him.

If you can't stay in hospital with your child, visit him as often as you can, and bring brothers and sisters to see him. Even if he cries when you leave, don't feel that he might settle better without your visits. It would only make him even more anxious, unhappy and abandoned. Make a special effort to be with him for the first day or two, and when he has any unpleasant procedures such as injections, or having his stitches removed.

WHAT TO PACK

These are general guidelines, as requirements vary from one hospital to another. Check with the ward sister before your child goes to hospital. Label everything, particularly toys.

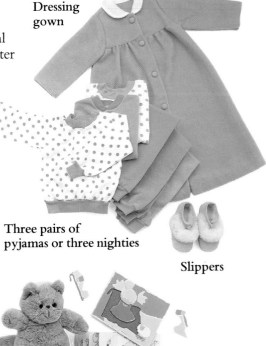

Dressing gown

Three pairs of pyjamas or three nighties

Slippers

Bib and feeding equipment

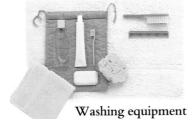

Washing equipment

Pack soap, a face-cloth, a sponge, her toothbrush and toothpaste, her brush and comb, and a towel.

Favourite toys

HAVING AN OPERATION

If your child is old enough to understand, it will help to explain what will happen on the day of his operation. Ask the doctor how the anaesthetic will be given (it may be injected or inhaled through a mask), and find out whether you will be allowed to stay with your child while he is given the anaesthetic. Try to be with him when he wakes up after the operation since he may be frightened.

1 Warn your child that he won't be allowed to eat or drink anything on the day of his operation.

2 Tell your child that he will be dressed up for the operation in a hospital gown, and will wear a bracelet with his name on it.

3 While he is still in the ward, your child will be given a 'pre-med' injection to make him sleepy.

4 Your child will be wheeled in his bed to the anaesthetic room, where he will be given an anaesthetic. He will fall asleep quickly.

5 If your child has stitches, discourage him from scratching them. It will hurt only momentarily when they are removed.

THE CHILD WITH A TEMPERATURE

In children, normal body temperature is between 36° and 37.5°C (96.8° and 99.5°F), depending on the time of day – it is usually lowest in the middle of the night and highest in the afternoon. A temperature above 38°C (100.4°F) may be a sign of illness. A child's temperature can shoot up alarmingly quickly when she is ill, but a slightly raised temperature is not a reliable guide to your child's health. Babies and children can be ill with a normal, or below normal, temperature, and some children can have a slight fever without being ill. So if your child seems unwell, she might be ill even if her temperature is normal. Her temperature may rise temporarily if she has been playing energetically, particularly in hot weather. If it is still above 38°C (100.4°F) after she has rested for about half an hour, she may be ill, so check for other signs of illness.

READING A THERMOMETER

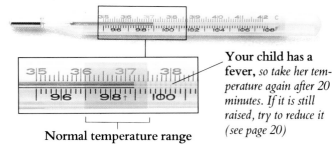

Call your doctor now: *your child has become dangerously chilled*

Your child has a fever, *so take her temperature again after 20 minutes. If it is still raised, try to reduce it (see page 20)*

Normal temperature range

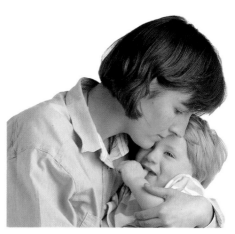

Feel your child's forehead with your cheek if you think he has a fever – don't use your hand because, if it is cold, your child's skin will feel warm by comparison. If his forehead feels hot, take his temperature.

■ SIGNS OF A FEVER ■

Your child may have a fever if:
- ▲ she complains of feeling unwell
- ▲ she looks pale and feels cold and shivery
- ▲ she looks flushed and her forehead feels hot.

■ CALL THE DOCTOR ■

Call the doctor now if your child:
- ▲ has a fever over 39.4°C (103°F) – over 38.3°C (101°F) if she is under a year old – and you can't bring it down
- ▲ has a fever for 24 hours.

CHOOSING A THERMOMETER

The best thermometers for babies and young children are the easy-read mercury thermometer, the digital thermometer and the temperature indicator strip. The easy-read thermometer contains mercury which, as it is warmed, expands up the tube alongside a temperature scale.

Safe and easy to use, the digital thermometer gives a quick and accurate reading. Although it is more expensive than other thermometers, it is ideal for young children. Always keep spare batteries.

Heat-sensitive panels on the temperature indicator strip glow in sequence and stop when they reach your child's temperature.

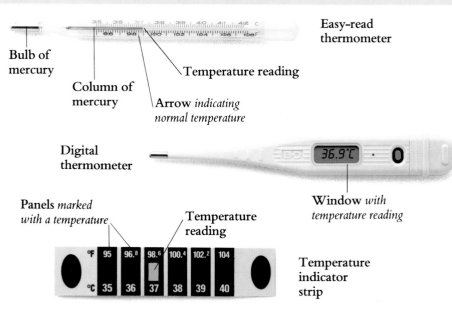

Bulb of mercury

Column of mercury

Arrow *indicating normal temperature*

Temperature reading

Easy-read thermometer

Digital thermometer

Window *with temperature reading*

Panels *marked with a temperature*

Temperature reading

Temperature indicator strip

TAKING YOUR CHILD'S TEMPERATURE

When your child is unwell, take her temperature at least twice a day, morning and evening. The best method is to place the thermometer under her arm, which gives a reading 0.6°C (1°F) lower than her true temperature. Never put a mercury thermometer into a young child's mouth, since it can break easily. The digital thermometer is not breakable, so it is safe to put it into a young child's mouth, but if she can't hold it correctly under her tongue, place it in her armpit, as for a mercury thermometer. The temperature indicator strip is much the easiest way of taking a young child's temperature, but the reading is less accurate than that of a thermometer.

USING A MERCURY THERMOMETER

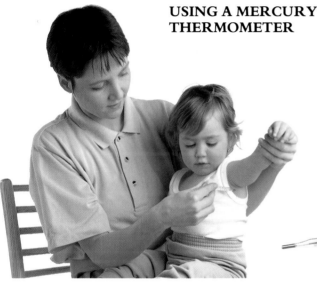

2 Bring your child's arm down and fold it over her chest. Leave the thermometer in place for the recommended time – usually about three minutes.

Hold the thermometer
firmly in place

3 Remove the thermometer and turn it until you can see the column of mercury next to the scale. Anything over 37°C (98.6°F) is a fever. Wash the thermometer in cool water, then dry it.

1 Hold the thermometer firmly and shake it sharply several times, with a downwards flick of your wrist, to shake the mercury back into the bulb. Then sit your child on your knee and lift her arm. Tuck the bulb end of the thermometer into her armpit.

The number
aligning with the top of the mercury column is your child's temperature

USING A DIGITAL THERMOMETER

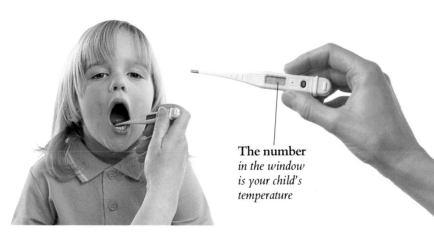

The number
in the window is your child's temperature

1 Switch the thermometer on and ask your child to open her mouth. Place the thermometer under her tongue and ask her to close her mouth. Wait for about three minutes.

2 Remove the thermometer and read your child's temperature. Anything over 37.5°C (99.5°F) is a fever. Switch the thermometer off, then wash it in cool water and dry it.

USING A TEMPERATURE INDICATOR STRIP

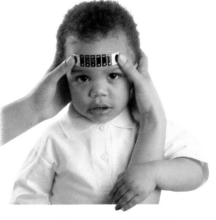

Hold the strip on your child's forehead for about 15 seconds. The highest panel that glows indicates your child's temperature. Anything over 37.5°C (99.5°F) is a fever.

BRINGING DOWN A FEVER

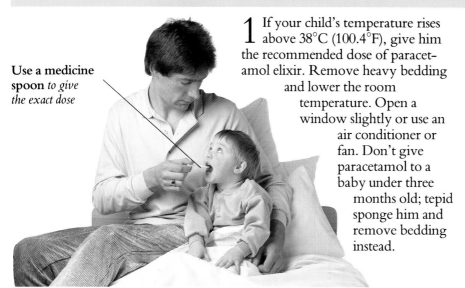

Use a medicine spoon *to give the exact dose*

1 If your child's temperature rises above 38°C (100.4°F), give him the recommended dose of paracetamol elixir. Remove heavy bedding and lower the room temperature. Open a window slightly or use an air conditioner or fan. Don't give paracetamol to a baby under three months old; tepid sponge him and remove bedding instead.

2 Your child will sweat profusely as his temperature falls, so give him plenty to drink, to replace the lost fluid. Change his bedding and pyjamas when his temperature is normal again, to make him comfortable.

TEPID SPONGING
If your child's temperature rises above 39.4°C (103°F), try to reduce it by sponging with tepid water as well as treating her as shown above. If your baby is under three months, just tepid sponge her.

1 Take off your child's bedding and remove her pyjama top. Put towels under her so that the bed does not get damp, then fill a bowl with tepid water and wring out a sponge in it.

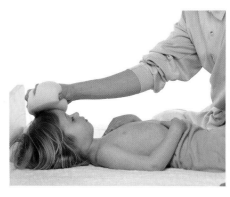

2 Gently wipe her face, neck, arms and legs. Let her skin dry naturally or allow an electric fan to blow gently on her. Continue for about half an hour, then take her temperature. If it is still above 39.4°C (103°F), **call your doctor now**.

FEVERISH CONVULSIONS
A rapid rise in temperature can cause a convulsion in a few children, making them lose consciousness and go rigid for a few seconds, then twitch uncontrollably.

What can I do?
Put your child on the floor and stay with her, but do not try to restrain her. Call your doctor as soon as the convulsion stops.

How can I prevent feverish convulsions?
If a tendency to have feverish convulsions runs in your family, keep your child's temperature as low as you can when she is ill. Follow the cooling methods shown above, and try not to let her temperature rise above 39°C (102.2°F). Your doctor may instruct you to give her a dose of paracetamol elixir when she shows the first signs of illness, to stop her getting a fever.

DELIRIOUS CHILDREN
Some children become delirious when they have a high fever. If your child is delirious, she will be very agitated, and may hallucinate and seem very frightened. This delirious state is alarming, but it isn't dangerous for your child. Stay with her to comfort her. When her temperature drops, she will probably fall asleep, and will be back to normal when she wakes up.

ALL ABOUT MEDICINES

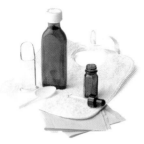

Most minor illnesses get better on their own, with or without treatment. Even if you have to consult your doctor, he may not prescribe a medicine. However, if a medicine is necessary, the doctor will tell you how often, and for how long, your child should take it. It is important to follow the directions carefully. Always shake the bottle before pouring out the medicine, and measure the dose exactly, using a medicine spoon. You can buy 5ml medicine spoons, droppers and tubes for giving medicine to babies, at most pharmacies. Never mix a medicine into your baby's feed or your child's drink, since he may not finish it. If your child struggles when you give him medicine or try to put drops into his nose, ears or eyes, ask another adult to hold him still while you give the medicine. You can prevent a baby wriggling by swaddling him firmly. If the doctor prescribes a course of antibiotics, your child must take the full course, even if he seems better before the medicine is finished, otherwise the infection may recur. However, antibiotics aren't effective against all illnesses: infectious diseases are caused by either viruses or bacteria, and antibiotic medicines destroy bacteria, but don't affect viruses. This means that there is no real cure for viral illnesses such as colds, measles, mumps and chicken pox – they simply have to run their course. Many other diseases, such as chest and urinary system infections, are caused by bacteria, and can therefore be treated successfully with antibiotics.

GIVING MEDICINE TO BABIES

When you give medicine to your baby, put a bib on him in case the medicine spills, and keep some tissues handy. Sterilize all the equipment in boiling water before giving medicine to a baby under six months. If your baby cannot yet sit up, hold him as if you were going to feed him. If he can sit up, sit him on your lap and tuck one of his arms behind your back. Keep your hand firmly on his other arm to prevent him struggling.

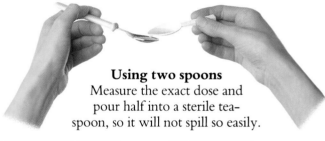

Using two spoons
Measure the exact dose and pour half into a sterile teaspoon, so it will not spill so easily.

MEDICINE SPOON

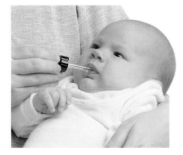

Measure your baby's dose and pour half into another spoon (see above). Keep both spoons nearby, then pick up your baby. Hold him so that he can't wriggle, then pick up one spoon and rest it on his lower lip. Let him suck the medicine off, then repeat with the rest of the dose.

MEDICINE DROPPER

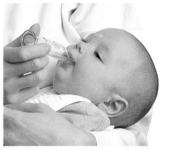

Measure the dose in a medicine spoon, then suck some of it into a dropper. Put the dropper into your baby's mouth and squeeze the medicine in. Give the rest of the dose. Don't use a dropper for a young baby: she could choke. Don't use a glass dropper if your baby has teeth.

MEDICINE TUBE

Measure the correct dose and pour it into the medicine tube, then pick up your baby and rest the mouth-piece of the tube on his lower lip. Tilt the tube slightly so that the medicine runs into your baby's mouth, but don't tilt it too much, or the medicine will run out too quickly.

FINGERTIP

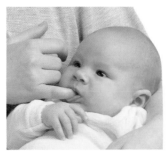

If your baby is reluctant to take her medicine, let her suck it off your finger. Measure the dose in a medicine spoon, then pick up your baby, keeping the spoon nearby. Dip your finger into it and let her suck the medicine off. Continue until she has taken the whole dose.

GIVING MEDICINES TO CHILDREN

Most medicines for children are made to taste fairly pleasant, but if your child dislikes the taste, the following tips may help.

■ Have your child's favourite drink ready to take away the taste of the medicine, and try bribery – a small treat or reward may help.

■ Tell your child to hold her nose so that she can't taste the medicine, but never do this forcibly for her.

■ If your child is old enough to understand, explain why she has to take the medicine – if she knows that it will make her feel better, she may be more inclined to take it.

■ If you really find it impossible to get the medicine down your child, ask your doctor if he can prescribe it with a different flavour or in a different form.

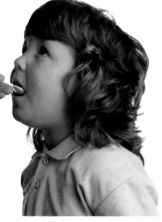

Giving medicine
If your child dislikes the taste of the medicine, pour it on to the back of her tongue – it won't taste so strong, since the taste buds are at the front.

■ MEDICINE AND SAFETY ■

Make sure that your child can't help herself to any medicines in the house.

▲ Keep all medicines out of her reach, preferably in a locked cabinet.

▲ Buy medicines with child-proof lids or packaging.

▲ Don't pretend to your child that her medicine is a soft drink.

Medicine and tooth decay
Clean your child's teeth after giving her medicine, because many medicines for children contain sugar. If your child has to take medicine for a long time, ask your doctor whether a sugar-free alternative is available.

■ WARNING ■

Never give aspirin to your child when she is ill; give her paracetamol elixir instead. A few children who have been given aspirin for a mild illness such as flu have developed a rare, but very serious disease called Reye's syndrome. If your child suddenly vomits and develops a high fever while she is recovering from an illness, **call for emergency help immediately.**

GIVING NOSE DROPS

CHILDREN

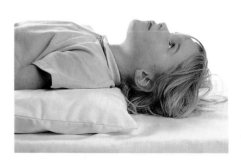

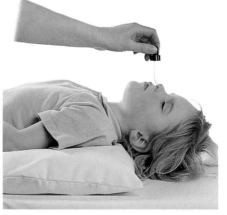

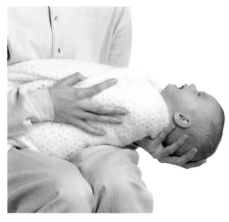

1 Place a small pillow or cushion on a bed and help your child to lie on her back with the pillow beneath her shoulders and her head dropped back. If your child is likely to wriggle as you give her the drops, ask another adult to help you by holding her head.

2 Put the tip of the dropper just above your child's nostril and squeeze out the prescribed number of drops. Don't let the dropper touch her nose – if it does, wash it before using it again. Keep your child lying down for about a minute.

BABIES
Swaddle your baby in a blanket, then lay her on her back across your knee, so that her head falls back over your left thigh. Put your left hand beneath her head to support it, then give the nose drops as instructed for a child.

GIVING EAR DROPS

CHILDREN

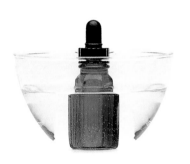

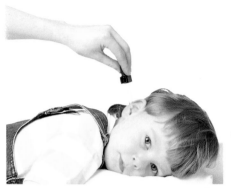

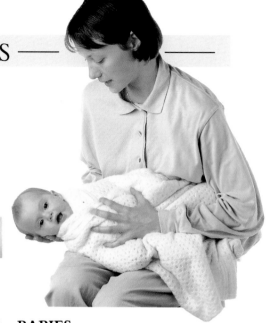

1 Most children find ear drops too cold as they go into their ears, so ask your doctor whether you can warm them up (some medicines go off if they are warmed). To warm them, place the bottle in a bowl of warm, not hot, water for a few minutes, then check the temperature on the inside of your wrist.

2 Ask your child to lie on his side with the affected ear uppermost, then place the dropper close to his ear and squeeze the prescribed number of drops into the ear canal. Keep your child lying down for about a minute and place a piece of cotton wool very lightly in his ear to prevent excess liquid running out.

BABIES
Swaddle your baby and lay her on her side across your lap with the affected ear uppermost. Support her head with one hand, then give the ear drops as instructed for a child.

GIVING EYE DROPS

CHILDREN

Hold your child's head *steady and pull her lower eyelid down gently with your thumb*

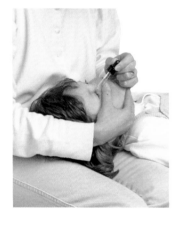

2 Hold the dropper over the gap between the lower lid and the eye, angling it so that it is out of your child's sight. If necessary, ask someone to hold her head steady. Squeeze out the prescribed number of drops, being careful not to touch the eye or the lid. Even if she cries, enough of the medicine is likely to stay in her eye.

BABIES
Choose a time when your baby is relaxed, then swaddle her and lay her on a firm surface or across your knee. Give the drops as for a child.

1 Bathe your child's affected eye with cotton wool dipped in warm boiled water, then ask your child to lie on her back across your knee or with her head in your lap. Put one arm round your child's head with your palm against her cheek, then tilt her head so that the affected eye is slightly lower than the other. Draw her lower eyelid gently down with your thumb.

EYE OINTMENT
If eye ointment has been prescribed, draw down the lower lid and squeeze in a thin sausage of ointment.

CARING FOR A SICK CHILD

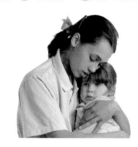

While your child is feeling ill, she is likely to demand a lot of attention, and may be irritable and easily bored. Most children become more babyish when they are ill, and both babies and children need a lot of extra cuddling and reassurance. Keep your baby with you during the day – let her sleep in her pram or carrycot, so that you can check on her frequently. Let your child lie down in the sitting room, so that she is near you. At night, sleep in the same room as your child if she is very unwell, so that you are nearby if she needs you. If possible, try to alternate with your partner, so that you have some nights of uninterrupted sleep. Many children vomit when they are ill, so keep a bowl nearby. Vomiting is rarely a serious symptom and, while it is often a sign of illness, it can also be brought on by emotional upset or excitement. Frequent or persistent vomiting can be a sign of a serious condition, and may lead to dehydration; see page 46 for when to call your doctor and how to prevent dehydration.

EATING AND DRINKING

Your child will probably have a smaller appetite than usual while she is ill. Because she is not running around as much, she will need less energy, so don't worry if she doesn't want to eat much for a few days – it won't do her any harm. Allow her to choose her favourite food, and offer small helpings. Let her eat as much or as little as she wants: when she is feeling better, her appetite will return. Babies may demand feeds more frequently than usual, but take very little milk each time. Be patient if your baby behaves like this – she needs the comfort of feeling close to you as she suckles.

Drink is much more important than food while your child is ill. Make sure that she has plenty to drink – about 1½ litres (3 pints) a day, especially if she has a raised temperature, or has been vomiting or had diarrhoea – to make sure that she doesn't get dehydrated.

Giving your child a drink
Let your child choose her favourite drink – it doesn't matter whether this is a fizzy drink, fruit juice, milk or water.

ENCOURAGING YOUR CHILD TO DRINK
If it is difficult to persuade your child to drink enough, make her drinks seem more appetizing by trying some of the ideas suggested below.

Small container
Offer frequent small drinks from a doll's cup or an egg cup, rather than giving large amounts.

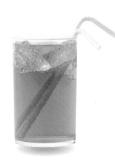

Straws
Make drinks look appetizing and more fun by letting your child use a straw.

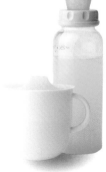

Teacher beaker
Offer drinks in a teacher beaker or bottle if your child has just grown out of either of these.

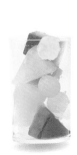

Ice cubes
For a child over a year, freeze diluted fruit juice into cubes, then let her suck the cubes.

Ice lolly
Your child may prefer an ice lolly – the 'drink on a stick'. Try to avoid ones with artificial colouring.

SICKNESS AND VOMITING

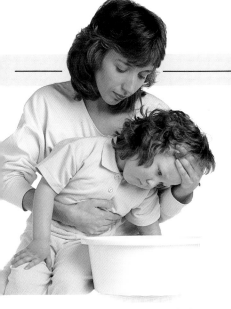

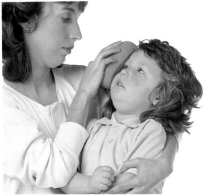

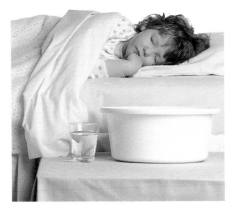

1 Hold your baby or child while she is vomiting to reassure and comfort her. Put a bowl nearby for her to be sick into. Support her head with one hand on her forehead, and put your other hand over her stomach, just below her rib cage.

2 After she has finished vomiting, reassure your child, then sponge her face and wipe round her mouth. Give her a few sips of water, let her rinse her mouth out, or help her to clean her teeth, to take away the unpleasant taste.

3 Let your child rest quietly after vomiting; she may want to lie down and sleep for a while. Wash the bowl and put it near her, in case she vomits again. If your child vomits frequently, she may have gastro-enteritis (see page 46).

COMFORT AND ENTERTAINMENT

STAYING IN BED

There is no need to insist that your child stays in bed, though if he is feeling very ill, he will probably want to stay there. If he wants to get up, make sure he keeps warm and that the room he is playing in isn't draughty. However, your child may want to lie down and go to sleep during the day, even if it isn't his usual naptime. If he doesn't want to be alone, let him snuggle with a pillow and a duvet on the sofa in the sitting room, or make up a bed for him wherever you are (a folding guestbed is ideal), so that your child still feels part of the family and does not get lonely.

Playing in bed

If your child feels like staying in bed, but wants to sit up, prop him up with pillows. Make a bed-table by resting a large tray or board on piles of books.

ENTERTAINING YOUR CHILD

Try to keep your child occupied, so that he doesn't get bored, but remember that he will act younger than his age while he is ill. He won't be able to concentrate for very long, and won't want to do anything too demanding. Bring out an old favourite toy he hasn't played with for a while. If you give him small presents to keep him entertained, don't be tempted to buy toys that are advanced for his age. Babies will enjoy a new mobile or a rattle that makes a new sound. Quiet activities such as interlocking building bricks, felt pictures, simple jigsaws, crayons or felt tip pens, a kaleidoscope, play dough or Plasticine are ideal for sick toddlers and children. Protect the bedding with a towel if your child wants to play with something messy while he is in bed.

COLDS AND FLU

All children get occasional colds and bouts of flu, and as soon as your child comes into contact with other children, he may seem to get one cold after another. Both illnesses are caused by viruses; as your child grows older, he will develop resistance to many of the viruses.

Wiping your child's nose
If your child has a runny nose, dab it gently with a tissue to prevent it becoming sore from frequent wiping. Throw the tissue away immediately, to avoid spreading the infection.

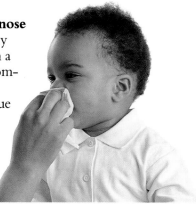

CALL THE DOCTOR

Consult your doctor as soon as possible if your child is under a year old, or seems very miserable and unwell, or has any of the following symptoms:
▲ temperature over 39°C (102.2°F)
▲ wheezy, fast or laboured breathing
▲ earache
▲ a throat so sore that swallowing is painful
▲ a severe cough
▲ no improvement after three days.

COLDS

What are they?
Perhaps the most common of all illnesses, a cold is an infection that causes irritation in the nose and throat. Children don't catch a cold simply by being cold – for example by going out without wearing a coat, or getting their feet wet. While it is not a severe illness, a cold should be taken more seriously in babies and children than in adults, because of the risk of a chest or ear infection developing. If your child develops a rash as well as the symptoms of a normal cold, she might have German measles or measles (see pages 29–30).

SYMPTOMS

▲ Runny or blocked nose and sneezing
▲ slightly raised temperature
▲ sore throat
▲ cough.

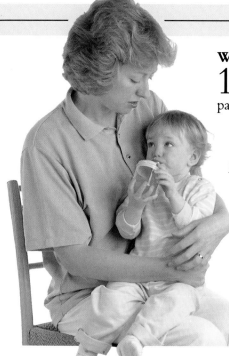

What can I do?
1 Take your child's temperature (see page 19), and give her paracetamol elixir to bring it down, if necessary. Make sure that she has plenty to drink, but don't force her to eat if she's not hungry. A drink before bedtime may help to keep her nose clear at night.

What might the doctor do?
If your baby has trouble feeding because her nose is blocked, your doctor may prescribe nose drops to be given just before a feed.

Nose drops and decongestants
Use these only if your doctor has prescribed them, and never use them for more than three days because if over-used, they can increase mucus production, which will make your child's nose even more blocked.

SINUSITIS
The sinuses are air-filled cavities in the bones of the face. The lining of the nose extends into them, so they can easily become infected after a cold. This infection, sinusitis, causes facial pain, but the sinuses that most often become infected don't develop until the age of three or four, so your child is unlikely to suffer from sinusitis before then.

FLU

What is it?

Flu (also known as influenza) is a very infectious illness caused by hundreds of different viruses. It tends to occur in epidemics every two or three years, when a new strain of the virus appears to which people have not yet developed immunity. If your child has caught flu, he will develop symptoms a day or two later, and will probably be unwell for about three or four days. He may feel ill enough to want to stay in bed for some of the time, and could feel weak for several days after his temperature goes down. A few children develop a chest infection such as bronchitis or pneumonia (see pages 42–3) after having flu.

SYMPTOMS

▲ Raised temperature
▲ headache
▲ aching all over the body
▲ shivery feeling
▲ runny nose
▲ cough
▲ sore throat.

What can I do?

Take your child's temperature (see page 19) and give him paracetamol elixir to reduce his fever if necessary. Make sure that he has plenty to drink, especially if his temperature is high. Offer your baby cooled boiled water.

QUESTION & ANSWER

"Should I have my child vaccinated against flu?"

If your child has a high risk of developing a chest infection after an attack of flu, a vaccination may be a good idea, so discuss it with your doctor. It will protect him from flu for about a year. However, since new strains of the virus develop every two or three years, the vaccine (which can only be made from existing forms of the virus) does not give life-long protection.

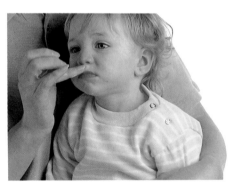

2 Smear a barrier cream, such as zinc and castor oil, under your child's nose and round her nostrils, if the area has become red and sore from a constantly runny nose or frequent wiping.

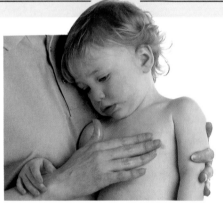

3 If your child is over a year old, rub a menthol chest rub on to her chest before she goes to bed.

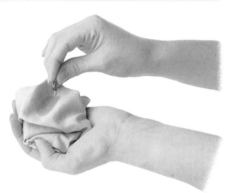

4 Sprinkle one or two menthol drops on to your child's night-clothes or a handkerchief. Tuck the handkerchief next to the mattress at the top of the cot or bed.

5 If your baby has a cold, she will be able to breathe more easily if you raise the head of the cot mattress slightly. Put a small pillow or a folded towel underneath it, then lay your baby in her cot so that her head and chest are slightly raised.

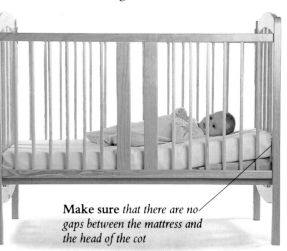

Make sure *that there are no gaps between the mattress and the head of the cot*

6 Keep your child's room warm, but make sure that the air isn't too dry, since breathing very dry air can be uncomfortable. Use a humidifier if you have one, or hang a wet towel near the heater in your child's room, to add moisture to the air.

HAVING YOUR CHILD IMMUNIZED

When your baby is about three months old, you should start the immunization programme which will protect her against most severe infectious diseases. When your baby is immunized, she is given a vaccine which contains harmless versions of the germ that causes the disease. The vaccine is too weak to cause the disease, but it makes the body produce special cells (antibodies) which will protect your child from that disease in the future. You must continue with the immunization programme even if your child catches the disease.

Why should my baby be immunized?

Some parents decide against immunization because they are worried about the possible risks or because they think that a disease is so rare that immunization is unnecessary. Unfortunately, once the number of children being immunized starts to drop, the disease can spread more quickly and easily, and epidemics start to occur. So by having your baby immunized, you are not only protecting her, but helping to eradicate the disease altogether.

What are the risks?

Immunization is safe, although it may make your baby mildly unwell for a short time. However, if your baby has had a convulsion, or has a close relative with epilepsy, she has an increased risk of a serious reaction to the whooping cough vaccine, so discuss this with your doctor. Do not take her to be immunized if she has a cold or is at all unwell, or has been taking antibiotics in the week before she is due to be immunized.

What are the after-effects?

Immunization may give your baby a slight fever, so keep a check on her temperature for 24 hours and, if it rises, give her the recommended dose of paracetamol elixir.

Your baby may develop a small, hard lump at the injection site. This will go in a few weeks, and is nothing to worry about. The measles vaccine may give her a rash and a fever up to ten days later, and the mumps vaccine might make her face swell slightly three weeks later. If she develops any other symptoms, or if her crying sounds unusual or her temperature rises above 38°C (100.4°F), **call your doctor now.**

Having an injection

Hold your baby firmly while she has the injection, to comfort her and keep her still. The doctor may inject her in the top of her arm or in her bottom or thigh.

IMMUNIZATION PROGRAMME		
Age	**Vaccine**	**How given**
Newborn	BCG	Injection
	OPV (Type 1)	By mouth
3 months	DPT	Injection
	OPV (Types 1, 2, 3)	By mouth
4–5 months	DPT	Injection
	OPV	By mouth
6 months	DPT	Injection
	OPV	By mouth
8–9 months	Measles	Injection
15 months	MMR	Injection
18 months	DPT	Injection
	OPV	By mouth
4–6 years	BCG	Injection
	DT	Injection
	OPV	By mouth

Key: DPT = diphtheria, pertussis (whooping cough), tetanus
OPV = oral polio vaccine
BCG (Bacillus Calmette Guerin) = tuberculosis
MMR = measles, mumps, rubella
DT = diphtheria, tetanus

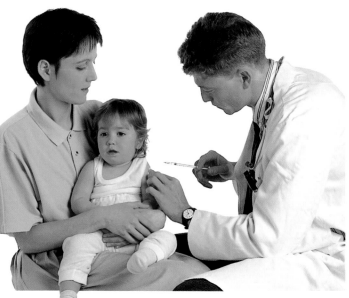

INFECTIOUS ILLNESSES

Now that most children are immunized, many of these diseases have become much less common. If your child catches one of them, he will probably be immune for the rest of his life. Since most of these infectious diseases are caused by viruses, there are no medicines to cure them (see page 21), but most children recover quickly and uneventfully. There is little point in trying to isolate your child when he has an infectious illness, unless he has German measles (see below), but it is a good idea to inform the parents of any children he has recently contacted.

WARNING

If your child has a raised temperature while he is ill with one of these diseases, **DO NOT** give him aspirin to bring the fever down, since it can cause a very serious disease called Reye's syndrome (see page 22). Give him paracetamol elixir instead.

EMERGENCY SIGNS

Call for emergency help immediately if your child has an infectious disease and develops any of these signs:
▲ unusual and increasing drowsiness
▲ headache or stiff neck
▲ convulsions
▲ rash of flat dark red or purplish blood-spots.

GERMAN MEASLES

What is it?
German measles is a very mild illness, so your child may feel perfectly well and may not want to stay in bed. She will develop symptoms two to three weeks after she has been infected.

What can I do?

1 Take your child's temperature at least twice a day (see page 19) and, if necessary, give her paracetamol elixir to reduce her fever.

2 Make sure that your child has plenty to drink, especially if she has a raised temperature.

SYMPTOMS

Days 1 and 2
▲ Symptoms of a mild cold
▲ slightly sore throat
▲ swollen glands behind the ears, on the sides of the neck and on the nape of the neck.

Day 2 or 3
▲ Blotchy rash of flat, pink spots appearing first on the face, then spreading down the body
▲ slightly raised temperature.

Day 4 or 5
▲ Fading rash, and general improvement.

Day 6
▲ Your child is back to normal.

CALL THE DOCTOR

Call for emergency help immediately if your child develops any of the emergency signs above. Consult your doctor as soon as possible if you think your child has German measles, but do not take her to the doctor's surgery in case she comes into contact with a pregnant woman.

What might the doctor do?
Your doctor will confirm that your child has German measles, but there is no treatment for it.

German measles and pregnancy
While your child is infectious, keep her away from any woman who might be pregnant. Although German measles is a mild disease, it can cause defects in a developing baby if a pregnant woman catches it.

MEASLES

What is it?

Measles is a very infectious illness which causes a rash, fever and a cough. Symptoms appear one or two weeks after your child has been infected.

Children usually feel uncomfortably ill with measles, and your child will probably want to stay in bed while her temperature is high. Some children develop complications such as pneumonia and ear infection.

SYMPTOMS

Days 1 and 2
▲ Runny nose
▲ dry cough
▲ red, sore, watering eyes
▲ raised temperature that gets steadily higher.

Day 3
▲ Slight fall in temperature
▲ continuing cough
▲ tiny white spots, like grains of salt, in the mouth.

Days 4 and 5
▲ Rising temperature – it may reach 40°C (104°F)
▲ dull-red rash of slightly raised spots appears, first on the forehead and behind the ears, gradually spreading to the rest of the face and trunk.

Days 6 and 7
▲ Fading rash and disappearance of other symptoms.

CALL THE DOCTOR

Call for emergency help immediately if your child develops any of the signs listed on page 29. Consult your doctor as soon as possible if you think your child has measles. Call him again if:

▲ your child is no better three days after the rash develops
▲ your child's temperature rises suddenly
▲ your child's condition worsens after she seemed to be getting better
▲ your child has earache
▲ your child's breathing is noisy or difficult.

What can I do?

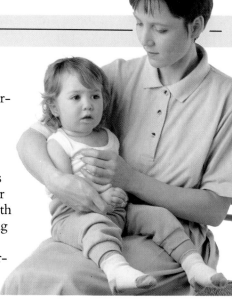

1 Check your child's temperature (see page 19) at least twice a day, and every five to six hours when her fever is high on days four and five. Stay with her if she is feeling very miserable while her temperature is high.

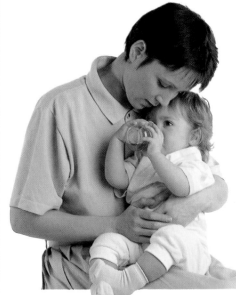

2 Make your child as comfortable as you can. Try to bring her temperature down with paracetamol elixir and, if necessary, by tepid sponging (see page 20).

3 Make sure that your child has plenty to drink, especially when her temperature is high.

4 If your child's eyes are sore, bathe them with cotton wool dipped in cool water. Although bright light won't damage her eyes, keep her room dark if this makes her more comfortable.

What might the doctor do?

There is no medical treatment for measles, but your doctor will confirm the diagnosis and may want to keep a check on your child until she has recovered. He will treat any complications if they develop.

CHICKEN POX

What is it?

This very infectious illness produces a rash of itchy spots. Your child may not feel very ill, but if she has a lot of spots, she may itch all over. Symptoms appear two to three weeks after your child has been infected.

The chicken pox virus causes shingles in adults, particularly the elderly, so keep your child away from old people while she is infectious.

SYMPTOMS

Days 1 to 9

▲ Crops of small, red, very itchy spots with fluid-filled centres, appearing in batches first on the child's chest, abdomen and back, later elsewhere on the body

▲ fluid within the spots becomes white and cloudy
▲ slight temperature
▲ the spots burst, leaving small craters
▲ scabs form over the spots and drop off after a few days.

Day 10

▲ Your child is back to normal, though some dried scars may still be present.

CALL THE DOCTOR

Call for emergency help immediately if your child develops any of the signs listed on page 29. Consult your doctor as soon as possible if you think your child has chicken pox, and call him again if your child has any of these symptoms:

▲ very severe itching
▲ redness or swelling around any spots, or pus oozing from the spots – this means they have become infected.

What can I do?

1 Take your child's temperature (see page 19), and give her the recommended dose of paracetamol elixir to bring it down if it is raised. Give her plenty to drink if she has a fever.

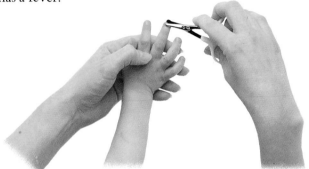

2 Try to discourage your child from scratching the spots, since it can infect them, and also cause scarring when they heal. Cut your child's fingernails short and keep them clean, so that the spots are less likely to become infected if she scratches them. Put scratch mitts on her.

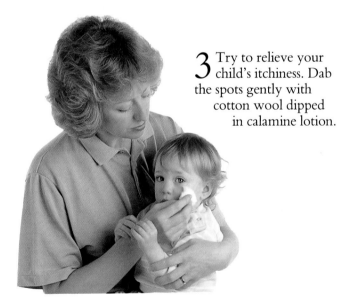

3 Try to relieve your child's itchiness. Dab the spots gently with cotton wool dipped in calamine lotion.

4 Give your child warm baths with a handful of bicarbonate of soda dissolved in the water, to help reduce the itching.

5 If your child is very itchy, she will probably find loose cotton clothes the most comfortable.

What might the doctor do?

Your doctor will confirm the diagnosis and may prescribe an antihistamine cream or medicine to relieve your child's itching if it is very severe. If any of the spots have become infected, he may prescribe an antibiotic cream.

MUMPS

What is it?

Mumps is an infection which causes swollen glands. It particularly affects the glands in front of the ears, making your child's cheeks look puffy. Your child will develop symptoms two to four weeks after he has been infected.

Occasionally, mumps causes inflammation of the testicles, but this is very rare in a boy before puberty.

■ SYMPTOMS ■

Day 1
▲ Pain when chewing, or facial pain that your child can't locate
▲ raised temperature.

Day 2
▲ Swelling and tenderness on one side of the face

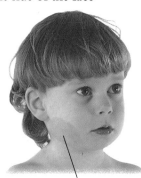

Area of swelling

▲ pain when opening the mouth
▲ raised temperature
▲ sore throat, and pain when swallowing
▲ dry mouth.

Day 3
▲ Increased swelling on the face, usually on both sides.

Days 4 to 6
▲ Gradual reduction of swelling and improvement in other symptoms.

What can I do?

1 Very gently feel your child's glands (see page 15) if he complains of pain in his face, or if his face looks swollen.

2 Check his temperature (see page 19) and give him paracetamol elixir to bring his temperature down if it is raised.

3 Encourage your child to have plenty of cold drinks, but avoid acidic drinks such as fruit juice. Let your child drink through a straw if it hurts him to open his mouth. Be patient when feeding your baby, since he may find sucking painful.

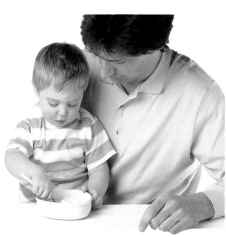

4 If it hurts your child to swallow, give him liquid or semi-liquid foods such as ice cream and soup.

■ CALL THE DOCTOR ■

Call for emergency help immediately if your child develops any of the signs on page 29. Consult your doctor as soon as possible if you think your child has mumps, and call him again if he develops bad stomach pain or a red testicle.

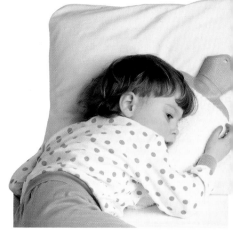

5 Fill a hot water bottle with warm water and wrap it in a towel, then let your child rest his cheek against it to soothe the swelling. Don't give a hot water bottle to a baby who is too young to push it away if it is too hot: heat a soft cloth and hold it gently against his face instead.

What might the doctor do?

The doctor will confirm that your child has mumps. There is no medical treatment, but your doctor will treat any complications if they develop.

WHOOPING COUGH

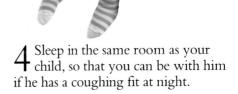

What is it?
One of the most serious childhood diseases, whooping cough is a severe and persistent cough. It is highly infectious, so keep your child away from babies and children who have not been immunized. Immunized children can get a mild form of the illness. A few children with whooping cough develop a secondary infection, such as bronchitis or pneumonia (see pages 42–3).

SYMPTOMS

Week 1
▲ Symptoms of a normal cough and cold
▲ slight temperature.

Week 2
▲ Worsening cough, with frequent coughing fits lasting up to a minute, after which your child has to fight for breath
▲ if your child is over about 18 months, he may learn to force breath in with a "whooping" sound
▲ vomiting after a coughing fit.

Weeks 3 to 10
▲ Cough improves, but may worsen if your child gets a cold
▲ your child is unlikely to be infectious after the third week.

What can I do?

1 Stay with your child during coughing fits, since he may be very distressed. Sit him on your lap and hold him leaning slightly forwards. Keep a bowl nearby so that he can spit out any phlegm he coughs up, and in case he vomits afterwards. Clean the bowl thoroughly with boiling water, to make sure that the infection doesn't spread.

2 If your child often coughs and vomits after meals, offer him small meals at frequent intervals, if possible just after a coughing fit.

3 Keep your child entertained – he will have fewer coughing fits if his attention is distracted, but don't let him get too excited or over-tired since this may bring on a coughing fit.

EMERGENCY SIGNS
Call for emergency help immediately if your child turns blue during a coughing fit.

CALL THE DOCTOR
Consult your doctor as soon as possible if you suspect that your child has whooping cough.

4 Sleep in the same room as your child, so that you can be with him if he has a coughing fit at night.

5 Don't let anyone smoke near your child, and don't give him any cough medicines.

What might the doctor do?
The doctor may prescribe a cough suppressant and an antibiotic. Although the antibiotic won't cure your child's cough, it may reduce its severity and make your child less infectious. This is particularly important if you have a baby who is at risk of catching whooping cough from an older brother or sister who already has the disease. However, the antibiotic is only really effective if it is given right at the beginning of the infection.

NURSING A BABY
Whooping cough is dangerous in babies because they may not be able to draw breath properly after coughing. Your baby will need careful nursing and may be admitted to hospital. She may find feeding difficult if she vomits frequently, so abandon your regular feeding schedule, and offer a feed as soon as she has calmed down after coughing or vomiting.

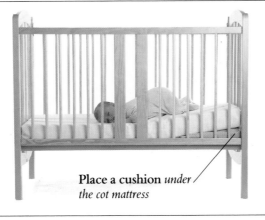

Place a cushion *under the cot mattress*

Coughing fits
When your baby has a coughing fit, lay her in her cot on her stomach with the foot of her cot slightly raised, or face down across your lap. Stay with her until she has stopped coughing and is breathing normally again. Cuddle her to comfort her after a bout of coughing or vomiting.

EYE PROBLEMS

Although most eye disorders clear up quickly when they are treated, all problems affecting the eye should be taken seriously. Eye infections spread easily to other people, so give your child her own face-cloth and towel, and change them frequently. Dry her eyes with tissues, using a clean one for each eye. Keep your child's hands clean and try to stop her rubbing her eyes – this helps to prevent an infection, as well as stopping it spreading.

■ EMERGENCY SIGNS

Call for emergency help immediately if your child has any injury which has damaged her eye, or if she cannot see clearly after an injury.

BLEPHARITIS

What is it?
Blepharitis is an inflammation of the edges of the eyelids, which usually affects both eyes. Many children with dandruff get blepharitis.

■ SYMPTOMS ■
▲ Red and scaly eyelids.

What can I do?
1 Dissolve a teaspoon of salt or sodium bicarbonate in a glass of warm boiled water, and use this to bathe your child's eyelids. Wash your hands before and afterwards, and use fresh cotton wool for each eye. Do this twice a day, making a fresh solution each time.

2 If your child has dandruff, wash her hair with an anti-dandruff shampoo. Use an anti-cradle cap shampoo for a baby.

■ CALL THE DOCTOR ■

Consult your doctor as soon as possible if:
▲ your child's eyes are sticky
▲ there is no improvement after about a week of home treatment.

What might the doctor do?
The doctor might prescribe a cream to soothe your child's eyelids, or an antibiotic ointment.

CONJUNCTIVITIS

What is it?
Also known as 'pink eye', because the white of the eye may turn pink, conjunctivitis is an inflammation of the lining of the eye and eyelids. It can be caused by a virus or by bacteria, being milder when it is caused by a virus. If your child's eyelids are gummed together with pus when she wakes up, she probably has bacterial, rather than viral, conjunctivitis. If your baby develops any of these symptoms in the first day or two of life, see Sticky eye, page 9.

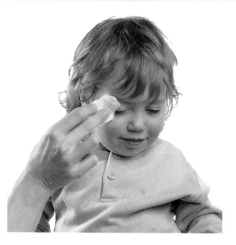

■ SYMPTOMS ■
▲ Bloodshot eye
▲ gritty, sore eye
▲ discharge of pus
▲ eyelids gummed together after sleep.

■ CALL THE DOCTOR ■

Consult your doctor as soon as possible if you think your child has conjunctivitis or if her eyes are bloodshot and sore.

What can I do?
1 Try to find out whether your child's symptoms might be caused by something other than conjunctivitis. She might have an allergy such as hayfever, or she may have a speck of dust or an eyelash in her eye. If she has an allergy, her eyes may be itchy and watering as well as red and sore.

2 If you think she has conjunctivitis, dissolve a teaspoon of salt in a glass of warm boiled water, and dip a piece of cotton wool in this. Bathe both of her eyes, using fresh cotton wool for each one. Start with the uninfected one, and wipe from the outside corner to the inside. Wash your hands before and afterwards.

What might the doctor do?
The doctor may prescribe antibiotic drops or ointment for a bacterial infection, which will cure it quickly. Viral conjunctivitis needs no treatment, but may last for a few weeks.

STYE

What is it?

A stye is a painful, pus-filled swelling on the upper or lower eyelid, caused by infection at the base of an eyelash. Some styes simply dry up, but most come to a head and burst within about a week, relieving the pain. Styes are not serious and you can treat them at home.

SYMPTOMS

▲ Red, painful swelling on the eyelid
▲ pus-filled centre appearing in the swelling.

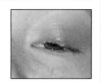

CALL THE DOCTOR

Consult your doctor as soon as possible if:
▲ the stye does not improve after about a week
▲ your child's whole eyelid is swollen
▲ the skin all round your child's eye turns red
▲ your child also has blepharitis.

What can I do?

1 Dip some cotton wool in hot water, squeeze it out and press it gently onto your child's stye, to help bring the stye to a head more quickly. Repeat this for two or three minutes three times a day until the stye bursts.

2 When the stye bursts, the pain is relieved. Wash the pus away very gently with cotton wool dipped in warm boiled water.

SQUINT

What is it?

Normally, both eyes look in the same direction at the same time, but in a child with a squint, one eye focuses on an object, while the other does not follow it properly.

A newborn baby's eyes do not always work together correctly, so intermittent squinting is common. This is nothing to worry about – your baby is simply learning to use his eyes. But if your baby's eyes don't move together after he is about three months old, he may have a squint.

Squinting may be constant or come and go. Children don't grow out of it, so treatment is essential. Delay may cause permanent weak vision in the squinting eye.

SYMPTOMS

▲ Eyes looking in different directions.

CALL THE DOCTOR

Consult your doctor if you think your child has a squint.

How can I check for a squint?

When your baby is about three months old, hold a toy 20cm (8in) from his face and move it slowly from side to side. Check that his eyes work together to follow the moving object.

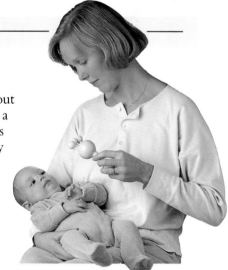

What might the doctor do?

The doctor will check your child's vision and may give him a patch to wear over his stronger eye for several hours each day, so that he is forced to use his weak or lazy eye. A toddler may need to wear glasses. If your child is under two, this treatment will probably cure his squint in a few months. If your child has a severe squint caused by muscle weakness, he may need to have an operation on one of the muscles in his weak eye, to correct the defect and straighten his eyes.

EAR PROBLEMS

Most ear problems in small children arise from an infection of the outer or middle ear, or because the tube connecting the ear and throat becomes blocked. Ear infections should be taken seriously, but they are dangerous only if they are not treated promptly: there is a risk that pus may build up behind the ear-drum, and eventually burst it, or that infection may spread into a bone behind the ear (mastoiditis).

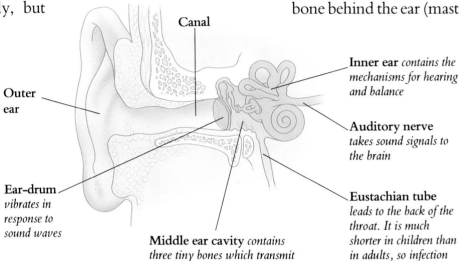

Canal

Outer ear

Ear-drum *vibrates in response to sound waves*

Middle ear cavity *contains three tiny bones which transmit sound signals to the inner ear*

Inner ear *contains the mechanisms for hearing and balance*

Auditory nerve *takes sound signals to the brain*

Eustachian tube *leads to the back of the throat. It is much shorter in children than in adults, so infection can spread easily*

Anatomy of the ear
Each ear consists of three parts. From the outer ear (the only visible part) a slightly curved canal leads to the ear-drum. Behind this is a cavity, the middle ear, in which lie three small bones, which transmit sound vibrations to the inner ear, the part of the ear that contains the structures concerned with hearing and balance.

OUTER EAR INFECTION

What is it?
The skin lining the outer ear canal becomes inflamed when your child has an outer ear infection. This may happen if he swims a lot in chlorinated water, or because he has poked or scratched his ear and it has become infected. Children with eczema are especially prone to such infections if they get water in their ears.

What can I do?
1 Give your child the recommended dose of paracetamol elixir to relieve the pain.

2 Make sure that water doesn't get into the affected ear at bathtime, and just sponge his hair clean. Don't let your child go swimming until the infection clears up.

What might the doctor do?
Your doctor will probably prescribe antibiotic or anti-inflammatory ear drops to clear the infection.

> ### SYMPTOMS
> ▲ Pain in the ear that is worse when the child touches his ear or lies on it
> ▲ redness in the ear canal
> ▲ discharge from the ear
> ▲ itchiness inside the ear.

> ### CALL THE DOCTOR
> Consult your doctor as soon as possible if you think your child has an outer ear infection.

WAX IN THE EAR

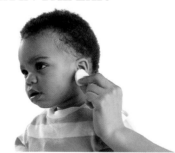

Wax sometimes accumulates in the ear, giving a feeling of fullness or partial deafness. If your child has a lot of ear wax, very gently wipe away any visible wax with cotton wool, but don't poke anything into the ear. If this doesn't help, consult your doctor.

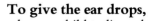

To give the ear drops, ask your child to lie on his side and keep still while you squeeze the drops into the affected ear. Keep him in this position for about a minute afterwards.

MIDDLE EAR INFECTION

What is it?
If your child has a middle ear infection, the cavity behind his ear-drum becomes infected or inflamed, usually because an infection has spread from the throat. The tube that runs from the throat to the ear is very short and narrow in a child, allowing infection to spread easily. Generally only one ear is infected. Once your child has had a middle ear infection, especially if this happens during his first two years, he is likely to have one in the same ear whenever he has a cold or throat infection.

SYMPTOMS

▲ Very painful ear, which may stop your child sleeping
▲ crying and rubbing or tugging at the ear, if your child can't yet talk well enough to complain of earache
▲ crying, loss of appetite and general signs of illness in young babies, especially after a cold
▲ raised temperature
▲ partial deafness.

What can I do?
1 Try to relieve your child's earache. Fill a hot water bottle with warm, not hot, water and wrap it in a towel, then let him rest his ear against it. Don't give a hot water bottle to a baby who is too young to push it away if it is too hot – heat a soft cloth and hold it against his ear instead.

2 If your child's ear is very painful, give him the recommended dose of paracetamol elixir.

3 If you notice a discharge, don't clear it away or probe his ear – just put a clean handkerchief over his ear. Encourage him to rest his head on the affected side, so that any discharge can drain away.

How can I prevent ear infection?
In cold weather, keep your child's ears warm. Use menthol drops or a menthol rub whenever he has a cold (see page 27). These help to clear your child's nasal passages, which reduces the chances of infection spreading to the ear.

CALL THE DOCTOR
Consult your doctor as soon as possible if your child's ear is infected or has a discharge.

What might the doctor do?
The doctor will examine your child's ears and may prescribe an antibiotic. If pus has built up behind the ear-drum, the doctor may prescribe a drug to help it drain away. If this is not effective, your child might need a small operation.

GLUE EAR

What is it?
Repeated middle ear infections can lead to glue ear, an accumulation of sticky fluid in the middle ear.

SYMPTOMS

▲ Partial deafness after repeated middle ear infections.

CALL THE DOCTOR
Consult your doctor as soon as possible if you think your child has glue ear.

What can I do?
Make an appointment to see your doctor if your child's hearing seems to be impaired after an ear infection.

What might the doctor do?
Your doctor may prescribe a decongestant, but a simple operation may be necessary. Under anaesthetic, a hole is made in the ear-drum and a tiny tube (a grommet) is inserted. The grommet is not uncomfortable, and will not affect your child's hearing, but he must not go swimming while it is in place. After several months it will fall out, the hole will heal, and his hearing will be back to normal.

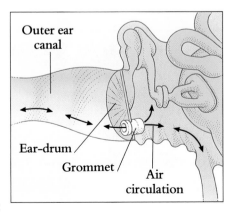

Outer ear canal
Ear-drum
Grommet
Air circulation

The grommet is implanted in the ear-drum, to equalize air pressure on either side of the ear-drum and to allow the ear to dry out.

MOUTH
INFECTIONS

A baby or child with a mouth infection will have a very sore mouth, so that feeding is painful. Thrush (see below) is the most common mouth infection in babies. Children over one are prone to cold sores (see page 54), usually on or around the lips, but sometimes inside the mouth.

Helping the child with a sore mouth

If your child's mouth is sore, try to make eating and drinking as painless as you can. Allow warm meals to get cool before giving them to your child, since hot food generally hurts more than cold, and offer her plenty of very cold drinks. If she is reluctant to eat or drink try some of the suggestions given here.

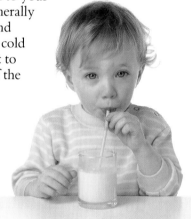

Let your child drink through a straw or
use a teacher beaker, since this may be less painful than drinking from a cup.

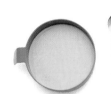

Soup This is nourishing and easy to eat, and can be served cold. Alternatively, liquidize food, or chop it very small.

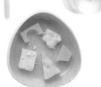

Cold drinks Serve drinks very cold, and avoid fruit juice, since it is too acidic.

Ice cream Your child may find cold food such as ice cream easy to eat.

Water

Cheese Encourage your child to finish meals with cheese and a drink of water to help keep her teeth clean without brushing.

THRUSH

What is it?

Thrush is an infection caused by a yeast which lives in the mouth and intestines. The yeast is normally kept under control by bacteria, but sometimes it multiplies out of control, producing a sore, irritating rash. Occasionally, it spreads through the intestines and causes a rash round the anus. It is not a serious infection and, although it does not respond to home remedies, it usually clears up quickly with medical treatment.

What can I do?

1 Wipe the patches in your child's mouth very gently with a clean handkerchief. If they don't come off easily, she probably has thrush. Don't rub them hard, because if you scrape them off they will leave a sore, bleeding patch underneath.

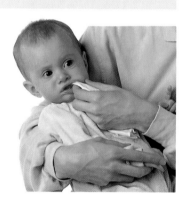

2 Give your child food that is easy to eat (see above). If you are bottle-feeding, buy a special soft teat and clean it carefully, then sterilize it after each feed.

3 If you are breast-feeding, continue to feed as normal, but take extra care with nipple hygiene to prevent your nipples becoming infected. Wash them in water only, not soap, after every feed, and don't wear breast pads. If they are sore or develop white spots, consult your doctor.

SYMPTOMS

- ▲ Reluctance to eat due to a sore mouth
- ▲ creamy yellow, slightly raised patches on the inside of the cheeks, tongue, or the roof of the mouth, which do not come away easily if you try to wipe them off
- ▲ in babies, a rash around the anus which looks like nappy rash.

CALL THE DOCTOR

Consult your doctor as soon as possible if you think your baby or child has thrush.

What might the doctor do?

Your doctor may prescribe a medicine to be dropped into your baby's mouth just before a feed, or, for a child over about two, lozenges to suck. If you are breast-feeding, the doctor may check your nipples for signs of infection.

THROAT INFECTIONS

S ore throats are common in children of all ages, and often accompany another illness, such as a cold or flu. Most mild sore throats clear up in a few days, but a more severe infection, particularly if your child's tonsils are affected, may give him a fever and make his throat so sore that swallowing is difficult and painful.

CALL THE DOCTOR

Consult your doctor as soon as possible if your child:
▲ has such a sore throat that swallowing is painful
▲ seems generally unwell and has a fever or a rash
▲ has infected tonsils
▲ has not been immunized against diphtheria.

SORE THROAT

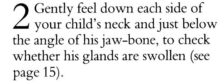

What is it?
A sore throat is an infection of the throat which makes the area sore and red. It may be part of a cold or flu (see pages 26–7), or one of the first signs of German measles or mumps (see pages 29 and 32). Children are prone to earache when they have a throat infection (see pages 36–7).

SYMPTOMS
▲ Reluctance to eat, because it hurts to swallow
▲ red, raw-looking throat
▲ earache (see pages 36–7)
▲ slightly raised temperature
▲ swollen glands
▲ stomach ache in young children.

What can I do?
1 Ask your child to face a strong light and open his mouth. Examine the back of his throat carefully (see page 15). If it is sore, it will look red and raw and you may be able to see creamy spots.

2 Gently feel down each side of your child's neck and just below the angle of his jaw-bone, to check whether his glands are swollen (see page 15).

3 Give your child plenty of cold drinks, and liquidize food if it hurts him to swallow. He may find very cold food such as ice cream less painful to eat than warm food.

4 Take your child's temperature (see page 19), and if it is above normal, give him the recommended dose of paracetamol elixir to bring his fever down.

What might the doctor do?
Most mild sore throats need no treatment, but if the doctor suspects that the infection is caused by bacteria, he may prescribe an antibiotic.

TONSILLITIS

SYMPTOMS
▲ Very sore throat
▲ red and enlarged tonsils, possibly covered with creamy spots
▲ temperature over 38°C (100.4°F)
▲ swollen glands on the neck.

What is it?
Tonsillitis is an inflammation of the tonsils, causing a very sore throat and other symptoms of illness. The tonsils are glands at the back of the throat, one on either side, which trap infection and prevent it spreading.

What can I do?
1 Examine your child's tonsils and feel his glands (see page 15). If infected, his tonsils will be large and red, and may have creamy spots.

2 Take his temperature (see page 19), and give him paracetamol elixir to bring it down, if necessary.

3 Encourage your child to have plenty to drink, especially if he has a fever. Offer him cold drinks and liquid or semi-liquid foods.

What might the doctor do?
Your doctor will examine your child's throat, and may take a throat swab by wiping a sterile swab across it. He may prescribe an antibiotic to clear the infection up quickly.

   If your child frequently has such severe tonsillitis that his general health suffers, your doctor may recommend that he has his tonsils removed. However, this operation is rarely done before a child is four.

COUGHS AND CHEST INFECTIONS

Most coughs in small children are a symptom of a cold or flu (see pages 26–7), which produces a dry, tickly cough. A cough may also be a symptom of a chest infection (see pages 41–3) or an early sign of measles (see page 30). A severe, persistent cough might be whooping cough (see page 33).

Your child may get a chest infection after having a cold or flu, if the infection spreads down towards his lungs. If he has a chest infection, he will have other symptoms as well as a cough: he may find breathing difficult, and might cough up some phlegm. However, slightly wheezy breathing is common in a small child with a cold or flu, because his airways are very narrow and become even narrower if they are swollen when he is ill, so this symptom on its own may not be a sign of an infection. Occasionally, a chest infection develops as a complication of measles or whooping cough.

■ **EMERGENCY SIGNS** ■

Call for emergency help immediately if your child:
▲ has a bluish tinge round his face, mouth and tongue
▲ is breathing very rapidly
▲ is breathing so noisily that it can be heard across the room
▲ seems to be fighting for breath
▲ deteriorates suddenly when he has a cold or flu
▲ is abnormally drowsy
▲ is unable to speak or make sounds as usual.

FREQUENT CHEST INFECTIONS

Babies under a year old and children with a long-term chest disorder such as asthma (see page 42) are prone to chest infections. If you smoke, your children are much more likely to develop chest infections than are the children of non-smoking parents.

If your child has frequent chest infections, your doctor may arrange for tests to find the cause.

Breathing
When your child breathes in, air is sucked down his windpipe and bronchi (the airways) into his lungs, where oxygen is absorbed into his bloodstream. His blood then carries the oxygen all round his body.

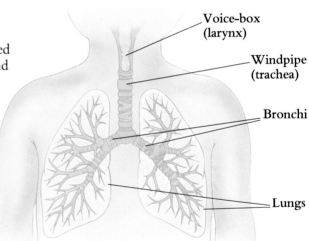

Voice-box (larynx)

Windpipe (trachea)

Bronchi

Lungs

CROUP

What is it?
Croup is an inflammation of the voice-box, which makes it swell, so that your child finds it difficult to breathe. Attacks of croup tend to occur at night, and usually last about two hours.

■ SYMPTOMS ■
▲ Breathing difficulty
▲ loud, crowing sound as breath is drawn in
▲ barking cough.

What can I do?
1 Keep calm, and reassure your child. He is likely to be very frightened, and if he panics, it will be even harder for him to breathe.

2 Create a steamy atmosphere by keeping a kettle boiling or taking your child into the bathroom and turning on the hot taps. The moist air will soothe his air passages and help him to breathe more easily.

3 Prop your child up on pillows, or hold him sitting on your lap – he will be able to breathe more easily in either of these positions.

■ CALL THE DOCTOR ■

Call your doctor now if your child has difficulty breathing, or if you think he has croup.

What might the doctor do?
The doctor will reassure you and tell you what to do if your child's croup recurs. He might prescribe an antibiotic, and may also give you some medicine to ease your child's breathing if he has another attack. If your child seems very ill, the doctor might send him to hospital.

COUGH

What is it?

A cough can be either a reaction to irritation in the throat or windpipe, or the result of a chest infection. A dry, ticklish cough is rarely serious. It probably means that your child's throat or windpipe is irritated, which may be a by-product of a cold, because mucus dribbles down the throat and irritates it. Her throat might also be irritated by smoke, if she is with adults who smoke. An ear infection can also cause a dry cough.

If your child has a moist-sounding cough, particularly if she coughs up phlegm, she probably has a chest infection. While most coughs like this are not serious, they can be a symptom of bronchitis or pneumonia (see pages 42–3).

■ CALL THE DOCTOR ■

Call your doctor now if, over a period of about half an hour, your child is breathing faster than usual, or if his breathing is laboured or very noisy. Consult your doctor as soon as possible if:
▲ your baby is under six months old and has a cough
▲ your child's cough prevents him sleeping
▲ the cough does not improve in three days
▲ your child has a recurrent cough.

What might the doctor do?

The doctor will examine your child and listen to his breathing. If your child has a dry cough, the doctor may prescribe a cough suppressant medicine to soothe his throat. If the cough is chesty, the doctor may carry out some diagnostic tests. He may prescribe antibiotics and perhaps a cough medicine to make the phlegm easier to cough up.

What can I do?

1 If your child has a sudden attack of coughing, check whether she might have inhaled a small object such as a sweet or a button. If she has, try to remove it (see Choking, page 66), but don't put your fingers down her throat to try to hook it out.

2 If your child has a chesty cough, try to help her clear the phlegm from her chest when she is coughing. Lay her on her stomach across your lap then pat her back rhythmically, but not too hard. Have a bucket or bowl nearby and encourage her to spit out any phlegm that she has coughed up.

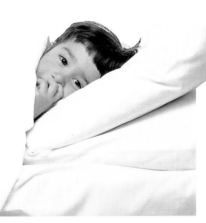

Keep your child's head *slightly tipped down*

3 Make sure that your child doesn't get cold while she has a chesty cough, otherwise the infection may spread further down into her chest, causing bronchitis.

4 If your child has a dry cough, give her a warm drink at bedtime to ease her throat. For a child over 18 months, make a soothing drink by dissolving a teaspoon of honey in a beaker of warm water and adding a few drops of lemon juice.

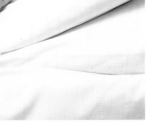

5 Prop your child up with extra pillows at night to help prevent mucus dribbling down his throat. For a baby, put a pillow under the head of the mattress.

6 If your child's cough is worse in a smoky atmosphere, don't let anyone smoke near him and keep him away from smoky areas.

7 Don't give him a cough medicine unless your doctor prescribes one.

BRONCHITIS

What is it?
Bronchitis is an inflammation of the lining of the main air passages leading to the lungs. It may follow a cold, flu or a sore throat because the infection has spread downwards.

Your child probably won't feel particularly ill, but he may have difficulty sleeping if his cough tends to be worse at night.

SYMPTOMS
▲ Rattly cough
▲ slight wheeziness
▲ slight temperature
▲ runny nose.

What can I do?
1 Help to relieve wheezy breathing and clear your child's lungs during a coughing fit. Lay him across your lap on his front and pat his back (see page 41).

2 Take your child's temperature and, if it is raised, give him paracetamol elixir, and plenty to drink.

3 Put a pillow under the head of your baby's cot mattress, to raise it slightly. When your older child goes to bed, prop him up with extra pillows (see page 41).

4 Until your child is better, keep him indoors in a warm, but not too hot or stuffy, room.

■ CALL THE DOCTOR ■
Call for emergency help immediately if your child shows any of the emergency signs on page 40. Consult your doctor as soon as possible if you think your child has bronchitis, and call him again if he:
▲ is no better after two days
▲ coughs up greenish-yellow phlegm.

What might the doctor do?
Your doctor might prescribe a cough suppressant to help your child sleep. If he thinks your child has a secondary infection, he might also prescribe an antibiotic to eliminate it.

ASTHMA

What is it?
Asthma is recurrent episodes of narrowing of the tiny airways leading to the lungs, which makes breathing, especially breathing out, difficult. It may be caused by an allergy, particularly if other people in your family have asthma, eczema or hayfever. Mild asthma is common, and your child will probably grow out of it.

SYMPTOMS
▲ Coughing, particularly at night or after exercise
▲ slight wheeziness and breathlessness, especially during a cold
▲ attacks of severe breathlessness, when breathing is shallow and difficult
▲ feeling of suffocation during an asthma attack
▲ pale, sweaty skin during an attack
▲ bluish tinge round the lips during a severe attack.

What can I do?
1 Keep calm and reassure your child. If he has had previous attacks, give him whatever medicine the doctor has prescribed. If this has no effect, **call for emergency help**.

2 Sit your child on your lap and help him to lean slightly forwards – this makes it easier for him to breathe. Don't hold him tightly – let him settle into the most comfortable position.

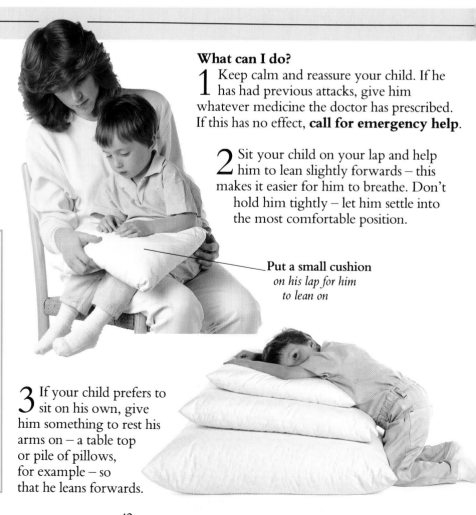

Put a small cushion
on his lap for him to lean on

3 If your child prefers to sit on his own, give him something to rest his arms on – a table top or pile of pillows, for example – so that he leans forwards.

PNEUMONIA

What is it?

Pneumonia is an inflammation of the lungs, which causes breathing difficulty. In young children it is nearly always due to the spread of an infection such as a cold or flu, and is usually caused by a virus, not bacteria. Occasionally pneumonia is the result of a tiny amount of food being inhaled into the lungs and causing a small patch of inflammation and infection.

Pneumonia is most common in babies under a year. Although it is a serious disease, most healthy babies recover completely in about a week.

■ SYMPTOMS ■

- ▲ Deterioration in a sick child
- ▲ raised temperature
- ▲ dry cough
- ▲ rapid breathing
- ▲ difficult or noisy breathing.

What can I do?

1 Prop your child up with extra pillows in bed, so that he can breathe more easily. For a baby, put a pillow under the head of the mattress.

2 Take your child's temperature and, if it is raised, try to reduce it by giving him the recommended dose of paracetamol elixir or tepid sponging him (see page 20).

■ CALL THE DOCTOR ■

Call for emergency help immediately if your child develops any of the emergency signs on page 40. Call your doctor now if you think your child has pneumonia.

3 Make sure that your child has plenty to drink, especially if his temperature is high. Offer your baby cooled boiled water.

What might the doctor do?

The doctor will advise you how to nurse your child, and, if the infection is bacterial, he may prescribe an antibiotic. If your child is very ill, he might need to be treated in hospital.

PREVENTING ASTHMA ATTACKS

Try to find out what causes your child's asthma attacks by keeping a record of when they occur. Vigorous exercise and over-excitement can bring on an attack. Some other common triggers are shown here.

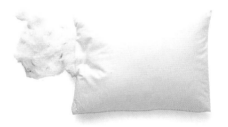

Feather-filled cushions or duvets
Change these for ones with a synthetic filling.

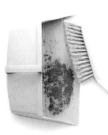

Dust
Reduce dust in your house by vacuuming and damp sponging, rather than sweeping and dusting. Cover your child's mattress with a plastic sheet.

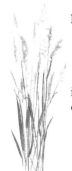

Pollen, especially from grass and trees
Discourage your child from playing in long grass, and keep him inside when the pollen count is high.

Animal fur If you have a pet, let it stay somewhere else for a while, and note whether your child has fewer attacks.

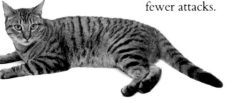

Cigarette smoke
Don't let people smoke near your child.

■ EMERGENCY SIGNS ■

Call for emergency help immediately if your child:
- ▲ has a bluish tinge on his tongue or round his lips
- ▲ is severely breathless
- ▲ does not start to breathe more easily ten minutes after taking his medicine
- ▲ becomes unresponsive.

■ CALL THE DOCTOR ■

Call your doctor now if this is your child's first asthma attack. Consult your doctor as soon as possible if you think your child may have asthma.

What might the doctor do?

The doctor may prescribe a drug to be given at the beginning of an attack, or before any activity which causes one. During a severe attack, he may send your child to hospital.

STOMACH PAIN

Pain between the bottom of the ribs and the groin, or "stomach pain", can be a symptom of many disorders, including gastro-enteritis (see page 46) and urinary system infections (see page 48). It may also be caused by vomiting, and can accompany illnesses such as tonsillitis and measles. Your child may complain of a tummy ache if he feels generally unwell or knows he is about to be sick, or if he has a pain somewhere else, but can't easily describe to you where it is.

DEALING WITH A TUMMY ACHE

What causes stomach pain?
Many children have recurrent bouts of stomach pain when something makes them feel anxious or insecure. Provided that your child's pain is not severe and lasts for only an hour or two, you needn't worry; try to find out what is bothering him, and reassure him.

However, if your child is in severe pain for a few hours, you should take it seriously. He might have appendicitis, when the appendix (a small, blind-ended tube attached to the intestines) becomes inflamed, though this is extremely rare in children under three.

Waves of severe stomach pain at intervals of about 15 to 20 minutes in a baby or toddler may mean that his bowel has become blocked.

What can I do?
1 Take your child's temperature. If it is slightly raised, he may have appendicitis, especially if the stomach pain is severe or seems to be located around his navel. Don't give him a pain-killer to ease it, or anything to reduce his temperature.

Wrap the hot water bottle *securely in a towel*

2 If you think your child may have appendicitis, don't give him anything to eat or drink. Otherwise, give him some water if he is thirsty, but don't let him eat anything.

3 Comfort your child by giving him cuddles and extra attention.

4 If you don't suspect appendicitis, fill a hot water bottle with warm, not hot, water and wrap it in a towel. Let your child lie down with this held against his stomach.

EMERGENCY SIGNS

Call for emergency help immediately if your baby or child:
▲ screams with pain at intervals of about 15 to 20 minutes, and goes pale when he screams
▲ passes dark red stools, or stools that resemble redcurrant jelly
▲ has severe stomach pain for longer than three hours
▲ has severe stomach pain combined with a raised temperature.

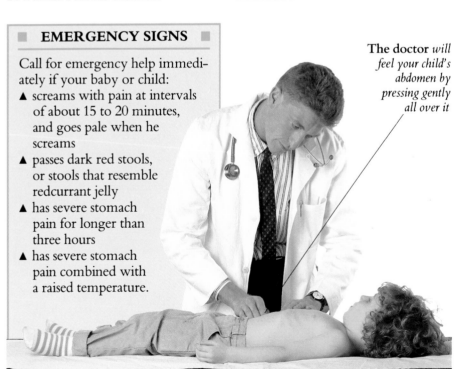

The doctor will feel your child's abdomen by pressing gently all over it

CALL THE DOCTOR

Call your doctor now if your child:
▲ develops any other symptoms
▲ has stomach pain for longer than three hours.
Consult your doctor if your child frequently has stomach pain.

What might the doctor do?
The doctor will examine your child to try to find out the cause of his stomach pain. The treatment will depend on his diagnosis, but stomach pain often needs no treatment. If the doctor suspects appendicitis or a blocked bowel, he will arrange for your child to go to hospital for an emergency operation.

CONSTIPATION, VOMITING AND DIARRHOEA

A minor change in diet can cause temporary constipation or diarrhoea. Vomiting or diarrhoea may accompany almost any illness, and can also be caused by excitement or anxiety. If your child vomits or has mild diarrhoea, check for other signs of illness (see pages 14–15). Frequent vomiting or severe diarrhoea can quickly make a baby or young child dehydrated. This is a serious condition, when the body loses too much fluid, and must be treated promptly (see page 46).

CONSTIPATION

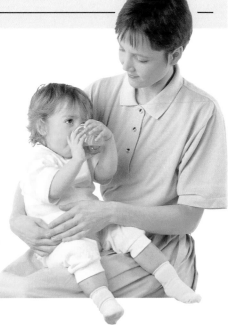

What is it?

If your child has constipation, she passes stools less frequently than usual, and they are harder than normal. Children's bowel habits vary greatly: some children have a bowel movement twice a day, others only once every two or three days. Whatever your child's regular pattern, it is quite normal – don't tamper with it. Babies quite often become slightly constipated when they learn to sit up or crawl, and before they can walk.

■ CALL THE DOCTOR ■

Consult your doctor as soon as possible if your child:
▲ cries or complains of pain when moving her bowels
▲ has streaks of blood in her stools or on her nappy or pants
▲ has constipation for more than three days.

What can I do?

1 Don't worry if your child is temporarily constipated, it won't do her any harm. Don't give her a laxative, since this will upset the normal action of her bowels, and don't add sugar to your baby's bottle.

2 Give your child plenty to drink, especially if the weather is hot, to soften her stools. Fruit juice may help to ease her constipation.

3 Don't hurry your child when she is on her potty, but don't leave her there for too long either. If she seems constipated, smear Vaseline around her anus before sitting her on her potty, to make her bowel movement easier.

4 Try to include more fibre in your child's diet (see below). This provides the bulk that helps the bowel to grip and move its contents along.

What might the doctor do?

The doctor may prescribe a mild laxative and give you some advice on your child's diet. If your child has streaks of blood in her stools, she could have a small tear in the lining of her anus, so the doctor may lubricate the area very gently.

GOOD SOURCES OF FIBRE

Some examples of foods rich in fibre are shown here. Fresh foods are always best. Wash vegetables and fruit well, remove pips and strings, and peel for a child under one year. Purée or mash the food for a baby under eight months.

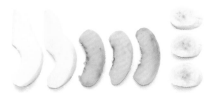

Fresh fruit Offer your child a variety of fruit such as slices of peeled pear, peach and banana.

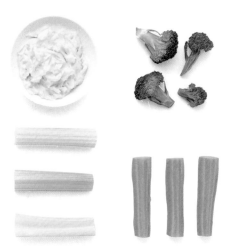

Fresh vegetables Mashed potato and lightly cooked broccoli are high in fibre. Celery and carrots can be served raw.

Wholemeal bread

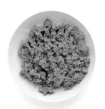

Wholemeal breakfast cereal

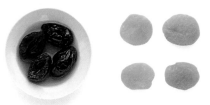

Dried fruit Prunes and apricots are ideal for young children.

VOMITING

What is it?
When your child vomits, she brings up most of the contents of her stomach. Babies under about six months old often regurgitate a small amount of their feeds. This is perfectly normal – your baby is not vomiting.

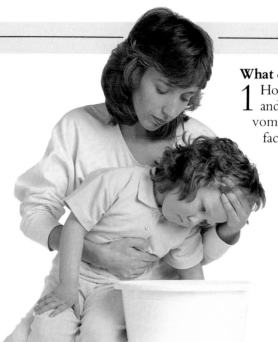

■ CALL THE DOCTOR ■

Call your doctor now if your child:
▲ vomits and seems abnormally drowsy
▲ brings up greenish-yellow vomit
▲ has vomited repeatedly for more than six hours
▲ shows any signs of dehydration.

What can I do?
1 Hold your child over a bowl and comfort her while she is vomiting (see page 25). Wipe her face afterwards and give her some sips of water.

2 Make sure that your child has plenty to drink – she needs 1 to 1½ litres (2–3 pints) a day. Make a glucose and salt drink (see Dehydration, below) and offer her a little every hour. If your baby won't take a bottle, try using a teaspoon or a medicine dropper (see page 21).

IDENTIFYING AND TREATING DEHYDRATION

Your child may be dehydrated if she shows one or more of the symptoms listed below:
▲ dry mouth and lips
▲ dark, concentrated urine
▲ no urine passed for six hours
▲ sunken eyes
▲ sunken fontanelle
▲ abnormal drowsiness or lethargy.

If your child is dehydrated, or is in danger of becoming so, make a glucose drink for her. Dissolve half a level teaspoon of salt and eight level teaspoons of sugar in a litre of water. Give her frequent drinks (30–60 ml every one to two hours) of this solution. Or buy oral rehydration powder from your pharmacy.

What might the doctor do?
The doctor will examine your child to find out what is making her vomit, and will then treat her according to the diagnosis.

If she shows signs of dehydration, the doctor may prescribe a powder to be added to her drinks. If she is very dehydrated, the doctor might arrange for her to be admitted to hospital, where she can be given liquid through a drip.

GASTRO-ENTERITIS

What is it?
Gastro-enteritis is an infection in the stomach and intestines which can be caused by germs or contaminated food. It is serious in babies, since it can dehydrate them very quickly, but it is rare in breast-fed babies. A mild attack in a child over two is not serious.

■ SYMPTOMS ■

▲ Vomiting and nausea
▲ diarrhoea
▲ stomach cramps
▲ loss of appetite
▲ raised temperature.

What can I do?
1 Make sure that your child drinks about 1 to 1½ litres (2–3 pints) a day. A glucose drink, made as described above, is best.

2 Don't give your child anything to eat until he stops vomiting, then introduce bland foods. Give your baby diluted feeds (see page 11).

3 Take your child's temperature and, if it is raised, give him a dose of paracetamol elixir to reduce it.

4 Let your child wear a nappy again if he has just grown out of them.

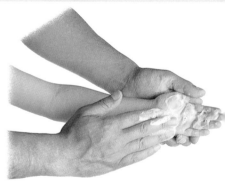

5 Make sure that your child washes his hands after using his potty and before eating. Wash your own hands after changing his nappy and before preparing his food. Sterilize all his feeding equipment.

DIARRHOEA

What is it?

If your child has diarrhoea, she will pass watery stools more frequently than normal. This may be the result of eating food that is too rich for her or that contains more fibre than she is used to.

■ CALL THE DOCTOR ■

Call your doctor now if your child:

▲ has had diarrhoea for more than six hours

▲ has blood in her stools

▲ shows any signs of dehydration (see left).

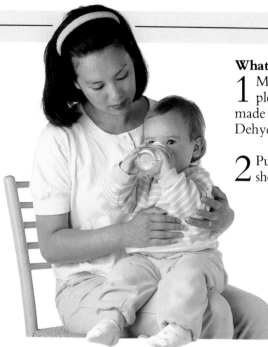

What can I do?

1 Make sure that your child has plenty to drink. A glucose drink, made as described for vomiting (see Dehydration, left), is ideal.

2 Put your child in a nappy again if she has just grown out of them.

3 Pay careful attention to hygiene: wash your hands after changing your baby's nappy and before preparing her food, and make sure that your child always washes her hands after using her potty and before eating.

What might the doctor do?

The doctor will examine your child to find out the cause of her diarrhoea, and will treat her according to the diagnosis. If your child has become dehydrated, the doctor may prescribe an oral rehydration powder to be added to her drinks. If she is very dehydrated, he might arrange for her to be admitted to hospital, where she can be given the extra liquid she needs through a drip.

ABNORMAL-LOOKING FAECES

Changes in the colour of your child's faeces are probably caused by a change in her diet, so check whether she has eaten anything unusual. Sometimes, though, an underlying illness accounts for the different appearance.

■ **Very pale, bulky faeces** that smell very offensive and float when you try to flush them away may mean that your child cannot properly digest gluten, a protein found in cereals (coeliac disease). Consult your doctor.

■ **Frothy, acid faeces** may indicate that your child can't digest milk properly (lactose intolerance). Consult your doctor.

■ CALL THE DOCTOR ■

Call your doctor now if your child:

▲ is under two and may have gastro-enteritis

▲ is over two and has had symptoms of gastro-enteritis for more than two days.

What might the doctor do?

The doctor will probably treat your child for dehydration and may advise you to give him only liquids for a few days. He may ask for a sample of your child's faeces.

QUESTION & ANSWER

"What steps can I take to prevent gastro-enteritis?"
Sterilize all your baby's feeding equipment for as long as he drinks milk from a bottle. Store made-up feeds in the main compartment of the fridge. It is important that they are never kept warm in a vacuum flask, since bacteria thrive in warm conditions.

Pay careful attention to hygiene when preparing food. If you store any cooked food, keep it in the fridge for no longer than two days, and make sure it is piping hot when you reheat it, because heat kills the bacteria that could give your child gastro-enteritis.

Wash feeding bowls and beakers in very hot water. Dry them on kitchen paper, not a teatowel.

If you are travelling abroad with a baby or small child, ask your doctor about any precautions you should take, particularly with regard to water, fruit and salads.

BLADDER, KIDNEY AND GENITAL PROBLEMS

Most urinary system infections are due to bacteria entering the urethra (see diagram below) and spreading up into the bladder. They are reasonably common in young children, and are usually not serious. Some children are born with minor abnormalities of the urinary system, which make them prone to such infections. Minor infections of the genitals are also quite common, and in babies and young children they are often part of the symptoms of nappy rash (see page 8).

The urinary system
Your child has two kidneys which filter his blood. The clean blood returns to his bloodstream, while the waste product (the urine) drains into his bladder, where it collects until he is ready to urinate.

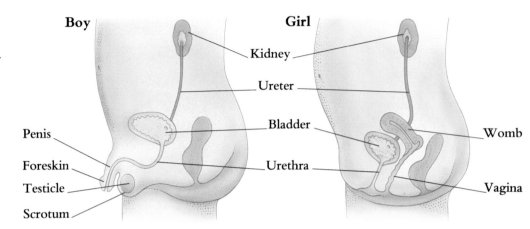

Boy — Girl — Kidney — Ureter — Bladder — Womb — Penis — Foreskin — Testicle — Scrotum — Urethra — Vagina

URINARY SYSTEM INFECTIONS

What are they?
Any part of the urinary system – the kidneys, the bladder and the connecting tubes – can become infected with bacteria. Infections are more common in girls, because the tube from the bladder (the urethra) is shorter in a girl than in a boy, and its opening is nearer to the anus, so germs can spread to it more easily.

What can I do?

1 If your child seems unwell, check to see whether her urine looks pink or cloudy. Note whether she is urinating more frequently than usual and whether it seems to hurt her to pass urine. If your child is still in nappies, you probably won't be able to tell that urination is frequent or painful, but you will probably notice a change in odour.

2 Make sure that your child has plenty to drink, to keep her kidneys flushed out.

3 Take your child's temperature and, if it is raised, give her the recommended dose of paracetamol elixir to reduce it.

SYMPTOMS
▲ Urinating more often than usual
▲ pain when urinating
▲ pink, red or cloudy urine
▲ change in odour of the urine
▲ raised temperature
▲ listlessness
▲ loss of appetite
▲ abdominal pain.

■ CALL THE DOCTOR ■
Consult your doctor as soon as possible if you think your child has a urinary system infection.

What might the doctor do?
The doctor will examine your child and may ask you to take a sample of her urine (ask your doctor how you should collect this). He may prescribe an antibiotic.

GENITAL PROBLEMS IN GIRLS

What can go wrong?
A little girl's vagina can become sore due to nappy rash (see page 8), an infection such as thrush (see page 38), or threadworms (see page 56). If your daughter has a blood-stained or smelly discharge from her vagina, she may have pushed something into it. Newborn girls often produce a white or blood-stained discharge for a few days, and this is nothing to worry about. After this age until just before puberty, a discharge is abnormal.

What can I do?
1 If your daughter's bottom is sore or red, don't use soap when you wash it – just use water, and dry it thoroughly. Always wipe from front to back, so that germs can't spread forwards from her anus.

2 Don't put plastic pants over your daughter's nappies, since they prevent air circulating to her bottom. If she no longer wears nappies, dress her in cotton pants, not nylon ones.

3 If your daughter has a discharge from her vagina, check whether she might have pushed something into it. If she has, **consult your doctor as soon as possible**.

What might the doctor do?
The doctor will examine your daughter and may take a sample of the discharge. If she has something lodged in her vagina, he will remove it gently. If she has an infection, he may prescribe antibiotics to be taken by mouth, or a cream to be applied to the affected area, depending on the cause of her symptoms.

SYMPTOMS
▲ Soreness or itching in or around the vagina
▲ redness around the vagina
▲ discharge from the vagina.

CALL THE DOCTOR
Consult your doctor as soon as possible if your daughter:
▲ has a discharge from her vagina
▲ still has symptoms after two days of home treatment
▲ has pushed something into her vagina.

GENITAL PROBLEMS IN BOYS

What can go wrong?
The foreskin, which covers the tip of the penis, can become inflamed or infected (balanitis), often as part of nappy rash (see page 8).

If a swelling develops in your son's groin or scrotum, he may have a hernia (a loop of the intestines bulging through a weak area in the wall of the abdomen).

What can I do?
If your son's foreskin is inflamed, wash it without using soap and dry it thoroughly at each nappy change, or at least once a day. Change to an enzyme-free washing powder and rinse his nappies or pants well.

How can I prevent inflammation?
Don't try to pull your son's foreskin back – it won't retract until he is at least four. If you try to force it, you may make his foreskin inflamed.

SYMPTOMS
Inflamed foreskin
▲ Red, swollen foreskin
▲ discharge of pus from the penis.

Hernia
▲ Soft, painless bulge in the groin or scrotum, which may disappear when your child lies down and get bigger when he coughs, sneezes or cries.

What might the doctor do?
If your son's foreskin is inflamed, the doctor may prescribe an antibiotic cream. If your son has a hernia, he may need no treatment, but if he is under six months old, or if the lump feels hard or does not disappear when he lies down, your doctor may recommend that he has an operation to repair the hernia.

CALL THE DOCTOR
Consult your doctor as soon as possible if:
▲ your son's foreskin looks red or swollen, or if there is any discharge
▲ your son's hernia becomes painful, or changes in any other way.
Consult your doctor if you think your son may have a hernia.

CIRCUMCISION
This is an operation to remove the foreskin. If you are thinking of having your son circumcised, discuss it with your doctor. Like any operation, it carries a small risk, so it is usually done only for religious or medical reasons.

SKIN PROBLEMS

Minor skin problems are common in childhood. Most clear up quickly, but some are very contagious, and must be treated promptly. If your child has a rash combined with other signs of illness, he may have an infectious illness (see pages 29–31). For other problems, see the guide below.

QUICK DIAGNOSIS GUIDE
One or more red spots, or a rash, see Spots and boils, Hives, Heat rash (below and opposite), Insect stings (page 76) or, if dry and scaly, see Eczema (page 52).
Raw, cracked areas, usually on or around the lips, or on the cheeks or hands, see Chapped skin (page 53).
Small blisters or crusty patches on or round the mouth, see Cold sores or Impetigo (pages 54–5).
Hard lump of skin, usually on the hands or feet, see Warts and plantar warts (page 54).
Itchy head, see Lice and nits (page 56).
Intense itching around the anus see Threadworms (page 56).

DEALING WITH ITCHING
Many skin problems cause itching, and since scratching can make the skin infected, it is important to relieve your child's itchiness.
■ Dress him in cotton clothes, since cotton is less irritating to the skin than wool or other fabrics.
■ Gently dab the area with cotton wool soaked in calamine lotion, to soothe inflamed or irritated skin.
■ Dissolve a handful of bicarbonate of soda in your child's bath.
■ Buy cotton scratch mitts for him to wear in bed.

SPOTS AND BOILS

What are they?
A spot is a small red swelling, usually on the face. A boil is an infection in the skin that causes a large, painful lump, which then festers to produce a head of pus in the middle. Boils are most likely to occur on the face or on pressure points such as the buttocks, but they can appear anywhere on the body.

Don't worry if your child gets occasional spots, but recurrent boils may be a sign of illness.

■ SYMPTOMS ■
Spot
▲ Small, red, painless lump.

Boil
▲ Painful, red lump which gradually gets larger
▲ white or yellow centre of pus appearing after a day or two.

■ CALL THE DOCTOR ■
Consult your doctor as soon as possible if:
▲ your child has a spot that looks inflamed
▲ your child has a boil in an awkward or painful place
▲ the centre of pus does not appear three days after the boil first developed
▲ red streaks spread out from the boil.
Consult your doctor if your child often gets boils.

What can I do?
1 If your child gets occasional spots, simply ignore them. They will clear up in a few days without treatment. If she tends to dribble, and the spots appear round her mouth, smear a barrier cream over the area.

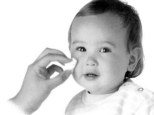

2 If your child has a boil, or a spot that looks inflamed, gently clean it and the skin around it with cotton wool dipped in antiseptic.

3 Cover it with sticking plaster. If it is rubbed by clothing, or is in a painful place such as on the buttocks, pad it with plenty of cotton wool then put sticking plaster over it.

4 The boil will come to a head and burst of its own accord in a few days. Don't squeeze it – this may spread the infection. After it has burst, clean it gently with cotton wool dipped in antiseptic, and keep it covered with sticking plaster until it has healed.

What might the doctor do?
The doctor may lance the boil and drain away the pus, to reduce the pain and swelling, and might prescribe a cream. If your child has a lot of boils, the doctor may prescribe a course of antibiotics.

HIVES

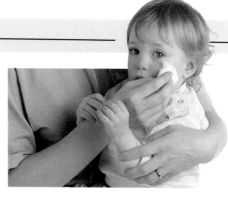

What is it?
Hives (also known as urticaria) is an itchy rash of red patches. The patches usually fade after a few hours, but new ones may appear. A nettle sting is the most common cause, but it can be caused by strong sunshine or by an allergy to certain foods or drugs.

■ SYMPTOMS ■

▲ Itchy rash of raised red patches (weals), sometimes with a pale centre
▲ weals varying in size from 1mm to 1cm ($\frac{1}{16}-\frac{1}{2}$in) across
▲ larger weals joining together.

What can I do?
1 Dab your child's rash with cotton wool dipped in calamine lotion.

2 If the rash is caused by an allergy, try to find out what your child is allergic to, so that you can help her avoid it in future. The rash usually develops a few hours after contact with an allergen, so try to remember whether, for example, she has recently eaten a new food.

■ CALL THE DOCTOR ■
Call your doctor now if your child's face, tongue or throat is swollen. Consult your doctor as soon as possible if:
▲ the rash does not disappear within four hours
▲ your child has frequent attacks of hives.

What might the doctor do?
The doctor may prescribe an antihistamine cream or medicine. He might also carry out tests to discover the cause of your child's allergy. If your child's face, tongue or throat is swollen, she might need an injection to reduce the swelling.

HEAT RASH

What is it?
Heat rash is a faint rash caused by overheating. It is more common in babies than in children, and usually appears on the face or in skin creases, where sweat can gather. It is not a serious disorder, and you can treat it yourself at home.

■ SYMPTOMS ■

▲ Pink rash on the face or in skin creases.

■ CALL THE DOCTOR ■
Consult your doctor as soon as possible if the rash has not faded 12 hours after your child cools down.

What can I do?
1 Take off any heavy bedding and remove a layer of your baby's clothing. Let him sleep dressed in just a vest and nappy.

2 Give him a bath in lukewarm water. Pat his skin dry gently, leaving it slightly damp so that he cools down as his skin dries. When he is dry, apply a little baby powder to absorb new sweat.

3 Take your baby's temperature and, if it is raised, give him the recommended dose of paracetamol elixir or tepid sponge him (see page 20).

How can I prevent heat rash?
Dress your baby in light clothes when the weather is hot, with cotton next to his skin, rather than wool or a man-made fibre. Keep him in the shade, or put a sun canopy over him.

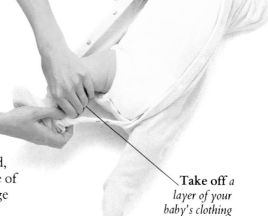

Take off *a layer of your baby's clothing*

What might the doctor do?
The doctor will check that the rash is just a heat rash. If it is, your baby needs no medical treatment. If the rash has another cause, the doctor will treat that.

ECZEMA

What is it?

Eczema is an allergy causing areas of itchy, red, scaly skin. It most commonly affects the face and skin creases such as the inside of the elbows and the back of the knees, but it can be more widespread.

It usually first appears between the ages of three months and two years, then improves as the child grows older. About half of all children with eczema grow out of it by the age of six, and nearly all of them grow out of it by puberty. Your child is more likely to develop eczema if other people in the family suffer from allergies such as eczema, asthma and hayfever.

SYMPTOMS

▲ Itchy, red, scaly, dry patches, usually on the face or in skin creases
▲ clear fluid oozing from the affected areas.

What can I do?

1 When you give your child a bath, clean the affected areas by wiping them with baby oil, rather than washing with soap. Rinse the oil off with plenty of water.

Use cotton wool *to apply the baby oil*

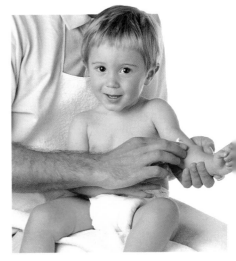

2 After a bath, apply an unscented moisturizing cream to your child's skin, since it may be very dry. Babies' brands are ideal.

3 Dress your child in cotton, rather than wool. In cold weather, put cotton clothing under warmer layers.

4 Try to stop your child scratching the affected areas – put scratch mitts on him at night if this seems to help, and keep his fingernails short.

5 Try to discover the cause of the allergy. Common allergens include foods (especially dairy produce and wheat), animal fur, woollen clothes and washing powder. Anxiety can trigger eczema, so find out if anything is worrying your child.

6 When your child's eczema is bad, keep him away from anyone with chicken pox or a cold sore.

CALL THE DOCTOR

Consult your doctor as soon as possible if:
▲ your child's eczema is very widespread or very itchy
▲ fluid is weeping from the eczema.
Consult your doctor if you think your child has eczema.

What might the doctor do?

The doctor may prescribe a cream, and if the area is infected, an antibiotic. If your child is allergic to a particular food, your doctor or clinic sister can advise you how to give him a balanced diet while avoiding that food.

SUNBURN

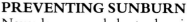

What is it?

Sunburn is sore or reddened skin caused by exposure to the sun. Babies and young children, especially those with fair hair and blue eyes, have very sensitive skin, so they are particularly vulnerable to it.

> ### ■ SYMPTOMS ■
> ▲ Red, sore areas of skin
> ▲ blisters appearing on badly affected areas
> ▲ flaking or peeling skin a day or two later.

What can I do?

1 Take your child inside or into the shade as soon as her skin begins to look red. Bear in mind that the worst symptoms of sunburn are likely to be delayed for a few hours.

2 Cool down any reddened areas of skin with cold water, then apply a soothing after-sun lotion or dab on some calamine lotion.

PREVENTING SUNBURN

Never leave your baby to sleep in the sun and, unless your child is used to the sun, don't let her spend more than 15 minutes uncovered in it at first, then increase the time by five minutes each day. Apply a sunscreen lotion every hour (choose one with a sun-protection factor of 10–15), and dress her in a T-shirt and a sun hat. Make her keep the T-shirt on when she is swimming or playing near water, to protect her shoulders. If her skin looks red the next day, keep her out of the sun.

> ### ■ CALL THE DOCTOR ■
> Consult your doctor as soon as possible if:
> ▲ your child has a fever and seems unwell
> ▲ blisters appear over a large area.

What might the doctor do?

The doctor may prescribe a soothing and healing cream.

CHAPPED SKIN

What is it?

Chaps are small cracks in the skin which occur when the skin becomes dry after being exposed to cold or hot, dry air. Chapping is not serious, but it can be painful.

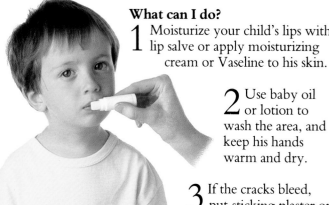

What can I do?

1 Moisturize your child's lips with lip salve or apply moisturizing cream or Vaseline to his skin.

2 Use baby oil or lotion to wash the area, and keep his hands warm and dry.

3 If the cracks bleed, put sticking plaster or surgical tape over them.

> ### ■ SYMPTOMS ■
> ▲ Tiny cracks in the skin, usually on or around the lips or on the cheeks or hands
> ▲ bleeding if the cracks are deep.

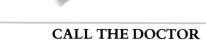

> ### ■ CALL THE DOCTOR ■
> Consult your doctor as soon as possible if:
> ▲ the cracks do not heal after three days
> ▲ the cracks become red and sore, or pus-filled.

What might the doctor do?

If the chapped area has become infected, the doctor may prescribe an antibiotic, otherwise there is no treatment.

COLD SORES

What are they?

Cold sores are small blisters, usually on or around the lips but they sometimes develop inside the mouth or elsewhere on the face.

They are caused by a virus which, once it has infected a child, lies dormant in the skin and tends to flare up occasionally, so if your child has had a cold sore, he is liable to get others in the future. Strong sunlight can trigger a recurrence, and so can a minor illness, such as a cold (which is why they are called cold sores).

What can I do?

1 At the first sign of a cold sore, hold an ice cube against the affected area for ten minutes. This may prevent the blister developing.

Wrap an ice cube *in a cloth and hold it against your child's lip*

2 If your child develops a blister, apply a soothing cream such as Vaseline.

3 Keep his hands clean, and stop him touching the sore, as he could spread the infection to his eyes.

4 Since cold sores are very contagious, don't let your child kiss other people and, if he tends to put toys into his mouth, don't let him share them with other children until the sore has gone.

SYMPTOMS
▲ Raised, red area that tingles or itches, usually around the mouth
▲ small, painful yellow blisters forming about a day later
▲ blisters crusting over after a day or two
▲ fever and general illness during the first attack.

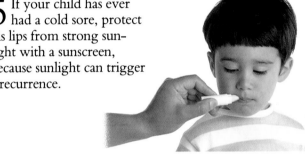

5 If your child has ever had a cold sore, protect his lips from strong sunlight with a sunscreen, because sunlight can trigger a recurrence.

CALL THE DOCTOR
Consult your doctor as soon as possible if:
▲ your child has a cold sore for the first time
▲ your child's cold sore starts to weep or spread
▲ your child has a cold sore near his eyes.

What might the doctor do?

The doctor will probably prescribe a cream to be smeared over the affected area several times a day, which will help the blister to heal.

WARTS AND PLANTAR WARTS

What are they?

A wart (verruca) is a lump of hard, dry skin; a plantar wart is a wart on the sole of the foot. They are caused by a virus that invades the skin. Almost all children get occasional warts or plantar warts.

Warts are not painful, and disappear spontaneonsly, so treatment is not necessary. Plantar warts are contagious, and tend to be painful because of the pressure put on them, so they should be treated promptly.

SYMPTOMS
Wart
▲ Hard lump of dry skin.

Plantar wart
▲ Hard, painful area on the sole of the foot, perhaps with a tiny black centre.

What can I do?

1 If your child has a wart, simply ignore it, unless it is on his genitals or by his anus. It will disappear on its own, probably after a few months, though some last for a year or more.

IMPETIGO

What is it?
Impetigo is a bacterial skin infection that may develop when a rash such as eczema or a cold sore becomes infected, though healthy skin can also become infected. It usually affects the skin around the mouth and nose, but can occur elsewhere. It isn't a serious disorder in children, but in a young baby it can spread and make him quite ill. It is very contagious, so prompt treatment is important. Untreated impetigo may be followed by a kidney disorder called nephritis. This is not common.

SYMPTOMS
- ▲ Rash of small red spots
- ▲ blisters forming over the spots
- ▲ the spots burst, then form large brownish-yellow crusts
- ▲ fever and general illness in a young baby.

What can I do?

1 Keep your child's face-cloth and towel separate from those of the rest of the family, and wash them frequently, so that the infection doesn't spread.

2 Try to stop your child touching the affected area – don't let him suck his thumb or pick his nose, as this could spread the infection.

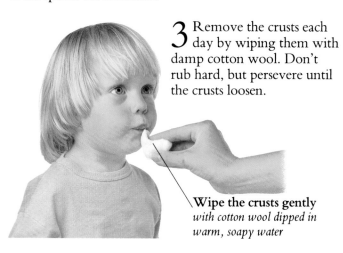

3 Remove the crusts each day by wiping them with damp cotton wool. Don't rub hard, but persevere until the crusts loosen.

Wipe the crusts gently *with cotton wool dipped in warm, soapy water*

4 Pat the area dry with a tissue or paper towel and throw it away immediately, so that the infection can't spread.

5 Keep your child away from other children, especially young babies, until he is better.

CALL THE DOCTOR
Call your doctor now if your baby is under three months old and suddenly develops widespread impetigo. Consult your doctor as soon as possible if you think your child has impetigo.

What might the doctor do?
The doctor may prescribe a cream and tell you to wipe the crusts away (see left) before applying it. If the infection is still there after five days, consult your doctor again.

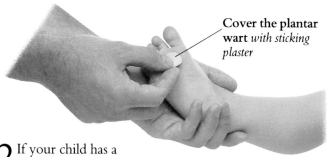

Cover the plantar wart *with sticking plaster*

2 If your child has a plantar wart, keep it covered with sticking plaster and don't let him go barefoot until it has cleared up. It may disappear spontaneously. Keep his towel and sponge separate from those of the rest of the family.

CALL THE DOCTOR
Consult your doctor if:
- ▲ your child's warts multiply
- ▲ your child has a wart on his genitals or anus
- ▲ your child has a plantar wart.

What might the doctor do?
Your doctor may prescribe a lotion to be painted regularly on to the wart or plantar wart until it disappears. Alternatively, he may refer your child to an out-patients' department at hospital, where it can be burnt or frozen off under local anaesthetic.

LICE AND NITS

What are they?

Lice are tiny insects which infest the hair, and make the child's head itchy. Their minute white eggs (nits) cling to the hair roots. Lice spread very easily from one head to another, so treat the whole family if your child picks up lice, and tell your friends to check their children's heads.

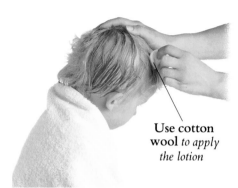

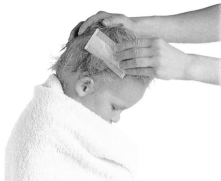

Use cotton wool *to apply the lotion*

| ■ | SYMPTOMS | ■ |

▲ Itchy head
▲ tiny white grains firmly attached to the hairs near the roots
▲ red bite marks under the hair.

What can I do?

1 Ask your pharmacist for a lotion to kill the lice and nits. Apply it all over your child's head, and leave it on his hair for as long as the instructions specify – usually several hours.

3 Clean your child's brush and comb, and his hats, in the lotion. Alternatively, seal his hats in a plastic bag and leave them for at least ten days – the lice and nits will all die.

2 Wash and rinse his hair, then comb it thoroughly with a special fine comb to remove the dead lice and nits. You may need to repeat this treatment two or three times, every three days, to eradicate the nits.

4 If your child goes to toddler group or playgroup, inform the staff that he has lice, and keep him at home until the lice and nits have been completely eradicated.

THREADWORMS

What are they?

Threadworms are tiny, white thread-like worms, about 1cm ($\frac{1}{2}$in) long. They can enter the body in contaminated food, and then live in the bowels, coming out at night to lay eggs around the anus, and causing intense itchiness. They are common in children, and are harmless, though the itching may be extremely uncomfortable. In little girls, the worms may crawl forwards to the vagina.

| ■ | SYMPTOMS | ■ |

▲ Intense itching around the anus, which is usually worse at night
▲ intense itching around the vagina
▲ tiny white worms in the faeces.

What can I do?

1 Try to prevent your child scratching, because she might inflame the skin around her anus or vagina.

2 Keep her fingernails short so that, if she scratches, she doesn't pick up any eggs under her nails, which could reinfect her or other people.

3 Make sure that the whole family washes their hands thoroughly after going to the lavatory and before eating. Use a nail brush to clean the nails properly.

| ■ | CALL THE DOCTOR | ■ |

Consult your doctor as soon as possible if you think your child has threadworms.

4 If your child no longer wears nappies, make sure she wears pyjamas, or cotton pants under a nightgown. Change her pants and pyjama trousers every day and sterilize them in boiling water to kill any worms or eggs on them. Change her bed-linen every day and wash and rinse it thoroughly in very hot water.

5 When she feels itchy, lay her across your lap and look for tiny white worms near her anus. Remove any you see with damp cotton wool and flush them down the lavatory.

What might the doctor do?

The doctor will probably prescribe a medicine for the whole family, which will kill the worms. He may also prescribe a cream for your child to soothe any inflammation around the anus or vagina.

EPILEPSY AND MENINGITIS

Although meningitis is rare, epilepsy (which causes convulsions) affects about one in 200 people. The most common cause of a convulsion in children is a high fever (see page 20), but this is not normally a form of epilepsy. Meningitis may develop as a complication of another illness.

EPILEPSY

What is it?
Epilepsy is a tendency to have seizures (also called fits or convulsions), which are bursts of abnormal electrical activity in the brain. With treatment, most children grow out of it by adolescence. There are several different types of epilepsy; two common forms in childhood are absence attacks and major seizures (see symptoms box).

What can I do?
1 Put your child on his side on the floor during a seizure. Stay with him to make sure he doesn't injure himself, but don't try to restrain him.

2 After a major seizure, put your child into the recovery position (see page 65). Don't wake him if he falls asleep, but make sure that he is breathing properly (see page 62).

3 Try to avoid letting your child get into situations that could be dangerous if he has a seizure – for example, put a guard at the top of the stairs, and don't leave him alone in the bath. But don't be over-protective – he shouldn't feel that his epilepsy makes him abnormal.

What might the doctor do?
The doctor may send your child to hospital for tests. He may also prescribe a drug to help control the seizures; if so, tell the doctor if your child's behaviour changes in any way, but don't stop giving him the drug.

> **SYMPTOMS**
>
> **Absence attacks (petit mal convulsions)**
> ▲ Sudden lack of movement
> ▲ dazed expression
> ▲ complete recovery in a few seconds.
>
> **Major seizures (grand mal convulsions)**
> ▲ Sudden unconsciousness, so your child falls down
> ▲ stiff arms and legs
> ▲ twitching or jerky movements
> ▲ urination
> ▲ sleeping, or gradual return to consciousness, when the twitching movements stop.

> **CALL THE DOCTOR**
>
> Call your doctor now if your child has:
> ▲ a major seizure for the first time
> ▲ a major seizure lasting more than three minutes
> ▲ a series of seizures in rapid succession.
> Consult your doctor if you think your child has absence attacks.

MENINGITIS

What is it?
Meningitis is an inflammation of the tissues that cover the brain. It is a very serious disease, and must be treated promptly. Inflammation of the brain itself (encephalitis) causes similar symptoms.

> **CALL THE DOCTOR**
>
> Call your doctor now if you think your child may have meningitis or encephalitis.

What might the doctor do?
The doctor may send your child to hospital for tests. His treatment will depend on the results of the tests, and he may need to stay in hospital until he has recovered.

> **SYMPTOMS**
>
> ▲ Fever
> ▲ listlessness and drowsiness, or sudden dramatic and uncharacteristic irritability or restlessness
> ▲ change for the worse in a child who has recently had an infectious illness such as measles or mumps
> ▲ vomiting
> ▲ loss of appetite
> ▲ headache or, in babies, slightly bulging fontanelle
> ▲ reluctance to bend the neck forward
> ▲ screwing the eyes up or turning the head away from bright light
> ▲ convulsions
> ▲ a rash of flat, dark red or purple blood-spots.

YOUR CHILD'S SAFETY

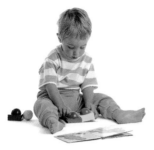

About a quarter of all the accidents that happen at home involve children under four, but there are a number of ways you can make your home safer. The best precaution of all is to keep your child under your own watchful eye. Remember that the chances of an accident happening are greatest when your child is tired, hungry or unwell, or when you are busy or worried. The risks are also high when the family is in a different environment – on holiday or away from home. When you buy equipment for your child, make sure that it has been approved by the South African Bureau of Standards (SABS), and use it only for the age of child it is designed for. Second-hand equipment should be sturdy and all the parts, including safety harnesses and brakes, must be in good working condition.

SAFETY IN YOUR HOME

ALL CHILDREN are accident prone, because their desire to explore and experiment far outstrips their common sense and forethought. Many accidents can easily be prevented, and it is your responsibility to make sure that your child can't injure himself. However, keeping him safe should not mean restricting his activities, but simply making sure that his world is safe for him to play in and explore.

Store polythene bags *and plastic wrap out of his reach*

Fit a guard *round your hob and turn your saucepan handles away from the front. Use the back rings rather than the front ones*

Fit a child-resistant *lock on your fridge or deep freeze*

Keep a gas, *foam or dry powder fire extinguisher*

Push hot drinks *to the back of kitchen surfaces*

KITCHEN
Your kitchen is full of potential hazards for your child and these dangers are increased if you are pre-occupied. So keep him away from the immediate cooking area when you are cooking – a bouncing cradle or a playpen is ideal. Remember that cooker rings, kettles and irons stay hot long after you have switched them off. At mealtimes, keep hot food and drink near the centre of the table, so that your child can't grab them. Don't use a table cloth, since he could pull it and spill hot things over himself. Make sure that your child can't get to your waste-bin.

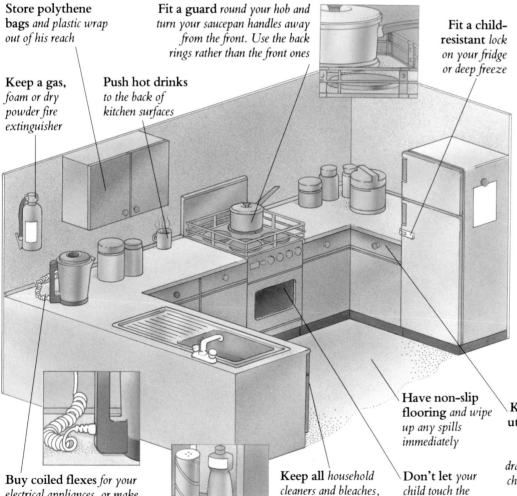

Have non-slip flooring *and wipe up any spills immediately*

Keep sharp utensils *such as kitchen knives in a drawer with a child-resistant catch*

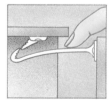

Buy coiled flexes *for your electrical appliances, or make sure that the flexes are short*

Keep all *household cleaners and bleaches, and your waste-bin, in a cupboard with a child-resistant catch*

Don't let *your child touch the oven door while it is hot*

KEEPING YOUR BABY SAFE

With each new skill your baby develops, he will find ways of running into danger, so think ahead to anticipate the possible hazards. He will learn to roll over when he is very young, so if you need to lay him down for a moment, put him on the floor. He will be able to grasp an object at about two months and reach for and grab things by about five months. Make sure that anything he can reach is safe to handle and too large for him to swallow or choke on. Don't eat, drink or carry anything hot, and don't smoke, while you are holding your baby. Never leave him alone with a bottle propped up in his mouth, since he could choke.

Always use safety straps on his pram, highchair and bouncing cradle, and don't put him in a bouncing cradle on a high surface because it could easily fall off.

Don't leave a young child alone with your baby: he might pick him up and drop him, or give him dangerous objects to play with.

BEDROOM

Your child will spend a lot of time in his bedroom, so make sure he can explore it safely. Don't put a pillow in his cot until he is at least two, and don't use loose plastic sheeting as a waterproof mattress cover. Never attach his toys to the cot with cords – they might wind round his neck. Keep large toys and cushions out of the cot – your child could use them as stepping stones to climb out – and don't string toys across the cot once he can stand. His toys should be made of non-toxic, non-flammable material, and must have no sharp edges or pieces small enough to swallow.

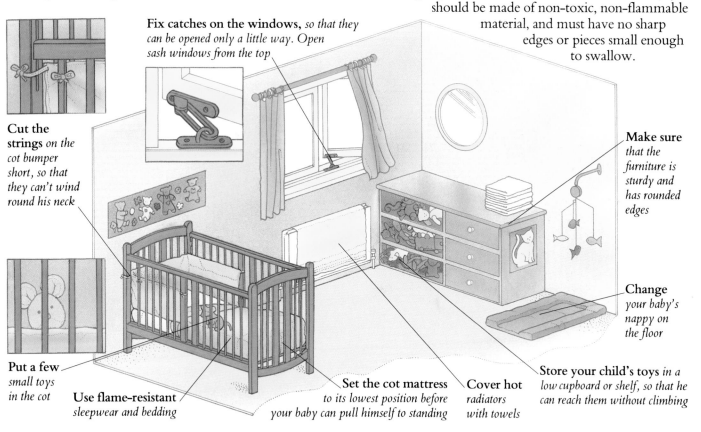

Fix catches on the windows, *so that they can be opened only a little way. Open sash windows from the top*

Cut the strings *on the cot bumper short, so that they can't wind round his neck*

Make sure *that the furniture is sturdy and has rounded edges*

Change *your baby's nappy on the floor*

Put a few *small toys in the cot*

Use flame-resistant *sleepwear and bedding*

Set the cot mattress *to its lowest position before your baby can pull himself to standing*

Cover hot *radiators with towels*

Store your child's toys *in a low cupboard or shelf, so that he can reach them without climbing*

BATHROOM

Never leave your child alone in the bath, even for a few seconds, until he is at least two-and-a-half, and use a non-slip bath mat. Set your water heater lower than 55°C (130°F), and run the cold water into your child's bath first. Test the temperature before putting your child in. Other accidents that may occur in the bathroom can easily be prevented:

■ Keep all medicines out of your child's reach in a cabinet with a lock or a child-resistant catch.

■ Put razors and cosmetics out of your child's reach.

■ Cover radiators and heated towel rails with towels.

■ If you have an electric heater, it should be wall-mounted, and have a pull-string switch.

■ Keep cleaning fluids and the toilet brush in a cupboard with a child-resistant catch.

■ If you have a shower with a glass screen, replace the screen with a curtain or install safety glass.

ELECTRICITY
Electric shocks from the mains can be very serious, so minimize the chances of your child receiving a shock:
■ Switch off electrical appliances when you are not using them.
■ Never leave a socket switched on with nothing plugged into it.
■ Cover unused sockets with dummy socket covers, or mask them with heavy insulating tape.
■ Check all flexes regularly, and renew those with bare wires.
■ Don't let your child play with toys powered from the mains until he is at least four.

LIVING ROOM
When you buy upholstered furniture, make sure that it will not give off toxic fumes if you have a fire. Fix a guard round all fires, and avoid using electric bar fires. Keep the television out of your child's reach, so that he can't touch the back.

Don't leave cigarettes, matches, alcohol, sewing equipment or coins lying around. Keep indoor plants out of his reach, as some are poisonous.

If you have low glass panels in doors or windows, use toughened, laminated or wire-net glass, or apply a transparent safety film, or put coloured stickers on them, so that your child can see where the glass is. Avoid glass-topped tables.

HALL AND STAIRS
Fix safety gates at the top and bottom of the stairs before your child can crawl or climb. Make sure that the hall, stairs and landings are well lit, and that your banisters aren't so wide apart that your child could fall through. Don't leave toys, piles of laundry, or anything else on the stairs. Make sure that the latch on the front door is out of his reach. It is a good idea to install a smoke detector.

Repair loose tiles or tears in rugs or flooring, and, if your floors are polished, fix a non-slip backing to any rugs. On polished floors, don't let your child wear socks without shoes, and make sure there are no splinters if you let him go barefoot.

GARDEN
Keep an eye on your child when he is playing in the garden, and if you leave your baby to sleep outside, put a cat net or an insect net over the pram. Never let your child play in or near a paddling pool without an adult supervising him, and empty the pool after use. If you have a waterbutt or a pond, cover it or fence it securely. Keep all your paths in good condition – remove moss and weeds regularly so that the paths don't become slippery, and repair them if they are uneven. Don't let your child play in an area where you have recently used pesticide, weed-killer or fertilizer.

CARS
Your child should always travel in a car seat that is officially approved for his age and weight. Use the child-proof locks on the doors so that he can't open them, and don't let your child lean out of the window or put his hand out while you are travelling.

Don't leave your child by himself in the car for more than a few moments, and when he is alone, make sure the handbrake is on, take the keys out of the ignition and leave the car in gear.

Check where your child is before closing the door or reversing your car – if he is just behind the car, you won't see him in the mirror.

Lock away *all your gardening and DIY tools, and any weed-killer, fertilizer and pesticide*

Teach your child *not to eat any berries*

Fix child-resistant *locks on all gates*

Make sure *that the plants in your garden aren't poisonous, and pull up mushrooms or fungi as soon as they appear*

Put your child's *play equipment on grass or sand, not on a hard surface*

Make sure *that the sand in your child's sandpit is too shallow for him to bury himself and teach him not to throw sand. Cover the sandpit when he is not playing in it*

FIRST AID

If your child is injured, always treat the most serious injury first. If he is unconscious, check his breathing, and resuscitate him if necessary (see pages 62–4), before giving first aid for any other injury. If he is breathing, first treat anything that might prevent him breathing properly, such as choking, suffocation or drowning (see pages 66–7), then control any heavy bleeding (see page 70). If your child is badly injured or in shock, he will need urgent medical treatment, but you should give first aid before calling for medical help. The instructions in this chapter explain how to cope with various injuries and tell you when help is necessary. If you need to get your child to hospital quickly, it may be faster to take him there yourself, rather than to call for an ambulance, but see below for occasions when you must call an ambulance.

GETTING YOUR CHILD TO HOSPITAL
Call for an ambulance, or ask someone else to phone if:
■ you think your child might have a spinal injury
■ you think he needs special treatment while travelling
■ you have no suitable transport of your own.
If you take your child to hospital yourself, try to get someone else to drive while you sit in the back with your child and continue to give first aid.

If you need an ambulance and your child is unconscious, don't leave him alone for more than a minute or so and, if you can, keep him in sight while you call for help. If he is not breathing, resuscitate him before phoning for an ambulance. Don't stop until he is breathing again, but shout to other people between breaths if necessary.

WARNING
If there is a chance that your child has injured his neck or spine – for example, after a bad fall – don't move him unless it is absolutely essential. Leave him in whatever position you found him while you check whether he is breathing. If you need to perform artificial respiration, get someone to help you if possible. Turn your child on to his back very gently without twisting his spine – try to hold his head, shoulders and hips, so that his body turns as a single unit.

FIRST AID KIT
Keep a supply of first aid equipment in a clean, dry container, and replace anything you use as soon as possible. Take some antiseptic wipes with you on outings, to clean cuts and grazes.

Surgical tape This is useful for sticking on dressings, and drawing together the edges of large cuts.

Cotton wool

Calamine lotion Soothes sunburn and insect bites and stings.

Eye bath

Non-adherent, absorbent, sterile wound dressings These peel easily off a wound.

One crepe bandage

Scissors

Tweezers

Triangular bandage This can be used to make a sling or secure a dressing.

Safety pins

Two gauze bandages

Prepared wound dressings These consist of a pad attached to a bandage, and are easy to put on.

Assorted adhesive plasters Use these for dressing minor cuts and grazes.

LIFE-SAVING TECHNIQUES

FAMILIARIZE YOURSELF with these instructions so that you can act quickly in an emergency. Every second counts. If your baby or child seems to be unconscious, follow these procedures before treating any injuries. If he has stopped breathing, it is vital to get air into his lungs quickly, so that he doesn't suffer brain damage. By breathing your own air into his lungs, you can prevent this, and revive your child. If his heart has stopped beating, you can pump it manually to keep his blood circulating round his body. Don't give up – children have revived after several hours of resuscitation.

> ■ **EMERGENCY** ■
>
> Call for emergency help if your baby or child becomes unconscious, even if this is only for a few seconds.

CHECKING FOR UNCONSCIOUSNESS

Tap the soles of your baby's or child's feet, and call his name. Note whether he responds.
Don't shake him, since this could worsen any injuries he may have.

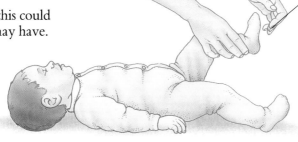

Tap *the soles of his feet*

✚ **If he doesn't respond,** he is unconscious, so check immediately that he is breathing.

✚ **If he responds,** check for injury and treat any he may have (see pages 66–77).

CHECKING BREATHING

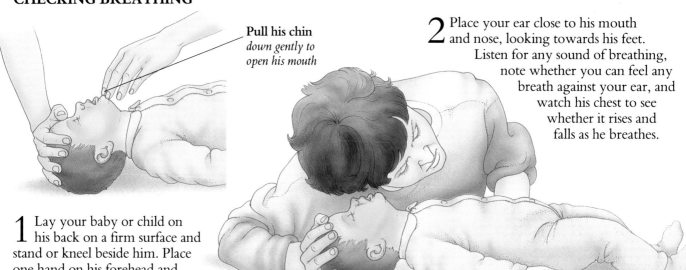

Pull his chin *down gently to open his mouth*

1 Lay your baby or child on his back on a firm surface and stand or kneel beside him. Place one hand on his forehead and press gently to tilt his head back slightly. Open his mouth.

2 Place your ear close to his mouth and nose, looking towards his feet. Listen for any sound of breathing, note whether you can feel any breath against your ear, and watch his chest to see whether it rises and falls as he breathes.

✚ **If there are no signs of breathing,** turn your child on to his side, or put him on his front over your lap. Sweep one finger round inside his mouth to clear any obstruction that might be blocking his breathing, but be very careful not to push anything down his throat. Check again for any signs of breathing.

✚ **If there are still no signs of breathing,** start artificial respiration straight away (see opposite).

✚ **If your child is breathing,** put him on his side in the recovery position (see page 65) and call for emergency help immediately.

ARTIFICIAL RESPIRATION FOR A BABY

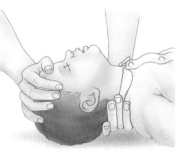

2 Take a deep breath, then place your lips round your baby's mouth and nose, making as good a seal as you can, then breathe out gently.

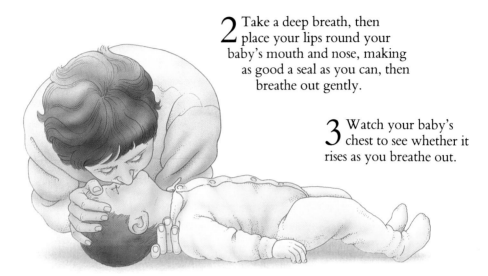

3 Watch your baby's chest to see whether it rises as you breathe out.

1 Slide one hand under your baby's neck, cupping the base of his head, to support him and keep his head tilted back. Leave your other hand on his forehead.

✚ **If his chest doesn't rise,** he probably has something blocking his windpipe. Treat him for choking (see page 66), then continue with artificial respiration if necessary.

✚ **If his chest rises,** remove your mouth from his face and let his chest fall. Give two quick, gentle breaths, then check his heartbeat (see next page).

ARTIFICIAL RESPIRATION FOR A CHILD

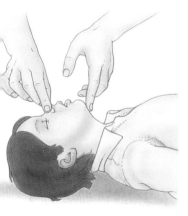

Pinch *his nostrils as you breathe into his mouth*

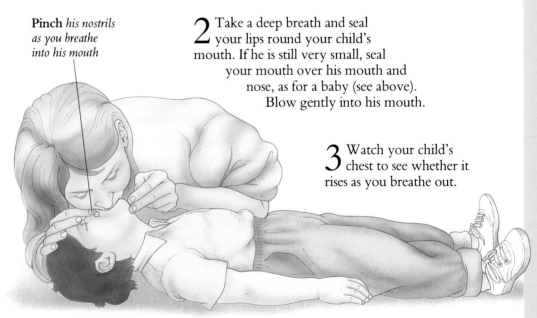

2 Take a deep breath and seal your lips round your child's mouth. If he is still very small, seal your mouth over his mouth and nose, as for a baby (see above). Blow gently into his mouth.

3 Watch your child's chest to see whether it rises as you breathe out.

1 Lift your child's chin to pull his jaw forward. Open his mouth and pinch his nostrils together.

✚ **If his chest doesn't rise,** he probably has something blocking his windpipe. Treat him for choking (see page 66), then continue with artificial respiration if necessary.

✚ **If his chest rises,** remove your mouth from his face and let his chest fall. Give two quick breaths, then check his heartbeat (see next page).

LIFE-SAVING TECHNIQUES *continued*

CHECKING HEARTBEAT

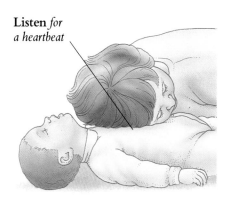

Listen *for a heartbeat*

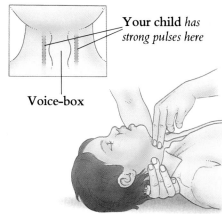

Your child *has strong pulses here*

Voice-box

For a baby

Put one ear gently against his chest and listen carefully for about five seconds to check whether you can hear a heartbeat.

For a child over two

Place the pads of two fingers over the voice-box at the front of his neck, then slide them into the slight hollow beside this. Feel for about five seconds.

For a baby or a child

➕ **If you can't feel a pulse or hear a heartbeat,** his heart has stopped. Start external chest compression immediately (see below).

➕ **If his heart is beating,** continue breathing gently into his lungs at a rate of about one breath every three seconds, until he starts to breathe on his own, or until emergency help arrives. As soon as he starts to breathe again, turn him on to his side in the recovery position (see opposite).

EXTERNAL CHEST COMPRESSION
For a baby

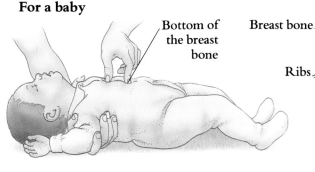

Bottom of the breast bone

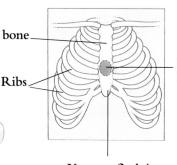

Breast bone

Ribs

Press here

You can find *the bottom of the breast bone by feeling where the rib-cage forms an inverted V-shape*

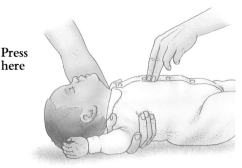

1 Slide one hand under your baby's shoulders and grasp the top of his arm. With your other hand, find the bottom of his breast bone (see right), then measure half-way up to his neck.

2 Place two fingers just below the middle of his breast bone and press down to a depth of about 1.5 to 2.5cm ($\frac{1}{2}$–1in), then release the pressure.

For a baby or a child

3 Give five compressions at a rate of about two per second, then give a breath into his lungs. Continue with five compressions followed by one breath until his heart starts to beat, or emergency help arrives. Every two or three minutes, check whether he is breathing and whether his heart has started to beat.

For a child over two

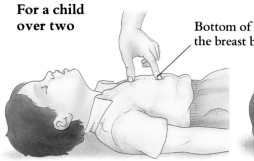

Bottom of the breast bone

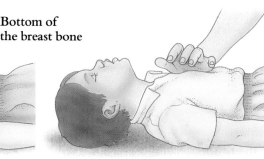

1 Find the bottom of your child's breast bone (see diagram above), then measure half-way up to the base of his neck.

2 Place the heel of one hand just below the half-way point and press down to a depth of about 2.5 to 3.5cm (1–1$\frac{1}{2}$in), then release the pressure.

4 When his heart starts to beat, stop giving compressions, but continue artificial respiration until he begins to breathe by himself, or help arrives.

THE RECOVERY POSITION

PUT YOUR BABY or child into this position if he is unconscious, but breathing. This is the safest position because it prevents his tongue falling back into his throat and obstructing his airway, and avoids the risk of him choking if he vomits.

1 Turn your child's face towards you, keeping his chin pulled forwards. Place the arm nearest to you by his side, and tuck his hand under his buttock, with the palm up. Fold the arm further from you over his chest, and cross his further leg over his near leg.

> **WARNING**
> Do not use the recovery position if there is a possibility that your child's neck or spine is damaged, for example, after a bad fall or a car accident.

His head *must be turned to one side and tilted well back with the chin jutting forwards*

2 Lay a coat or blanket in front of your child, if available. Put one hand by his face to protect it, then grasp his hip with your other hand. Roll him towards you on to the coat or blanket.

3 Make sure that his nose and mouth aren't obstructed, then bend his top arm and leg up to a right angle, so that they support him. Gently pull his lower arm out from under his hip, and leave it by his side.

4 Cover him with a coat or blanket, then call for emergency help. Stay with him until help arrives, and every three minutes check his breathing and his heartbeat (see opposite), if his heart had stopped.

CHOKING

This happens when a small object or piece of food gets lodged in the windpipe, causing a coughing fit. It is important to dislodge the object quickly, so that your child can breathe properly again. Choking is common in very young children, who tend to put everything they get hold of into their mouths. They may find it hard to swallow dry, crumbly foods, so avoid them if possible.

HELPING A BABY

1 Hold your baby face down with his head lower than his body: either support him along your forearm, or hold him upside down by his ankles. Strike him between the shoulder-blades up to four times.

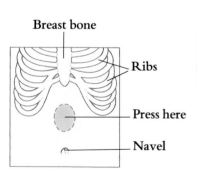

Breast bone

Ribs

Press here

Navel

2 If he is still choking, lay him on his side and tilt his head back slightly. Support his back with one hand, and place two fingers of your other hand about half-way between his navel and the point where the bottom of his ribs forms an inverted V-shape (see diagram). Press inwards and upwards with a quick, thrusting movement.

3 If your baby does not start breathing normally when the blockage is removed, carry out artificial respiration immediately (see pages 63–4).

HELPING A CHILD

1 Sit down or kneel on one knee and lay your child on her front over your knee, with her head hanging down. Support her chest with one hand and strike her between her shoulder-blades several times.

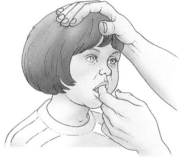

2 If this fails to dislodge the obstruction, sweep around your child's mouth with a finger and try to hook it from the back of her throat. Be very careful not to push anything further down her throat.

3 If she is still choking, sit her on your lap, facing forwards. Support her back with one hand and hold the other in a fist, thumb inwards, half-way between her navel and the V-shape at the bottom of her ribs (see diagram, left). Press sharply inwards and upwards, up to four times.

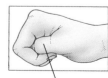

Tuck your thumb in *when you make a fist*

4 If your child does not start breathing normally when the blockage is removed, carry out artificial respiration (see pages 63–4).

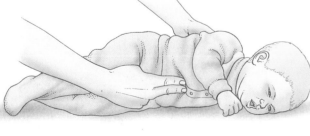

SUFFOCATION

Anything lying across your child's face may block her mouth and nose, and prevent her breathing.

What can I do?

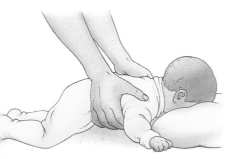

| ■ | **EMERGENCY** | ■ |

Call for emergency help immediately if your child:
▲ becomes unconscious
▲ stops breathing, even if only for a few seconds
▲ shows any symptoms that worry you.

1 Pick your child up or remove whatever is covering her face.

2 Check whether your child is conscious and breathing (see page 62).

✚ **If she is not breathing,** start artificial respiration immediately (see pages 63–4) and ask someone to call for emergency help.

✚ **If she is breathing but unconscious,** place her in the recovery position (see page 65), then call for emergency help.

✚ **If she is conscious,** simply comfort and reassure her.

DROWNING

Babies and children can drown in very shallow water. When a young child's face is submerged, his automatic reaction is to take a deep breath to scream, rather than to lift his face clear of the water.

What can I do?
Check whether your child is conscious and breathing (see page 62). If he is coughing, choking, or vomiting, he is still breathing. If there is any chance that he has injured his neck or back, lift him very gently and make sure that you don't twist his spine.

✚ **If he is not breathing,** don't waste time trying to drain the water from his lungs. Clear any debris, such as mud or seaweed, from his mouth and start artificial respiration (see pages 63–4) straight away – if possible while he is still being carried from the water – and **call for emergency help.** Continue artificial respiration until help arrives or until he starts to breathe again. When he starts to breathe again, put him in the recovery position (see page 65).

| ■ | **EMERGENCY** | ■ |

Call for emergency help immediately if your child was rescued from drowning, even if he didn't become unconscious.

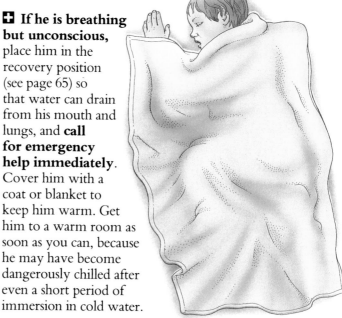

✚ **If he is breathing but unconscious,** place him in the recovery position (see page 65) so that water can drain from his mouth and lungs, and **call for emergency help immediately.** Cover him with a coat or blanket to keep him warm. Get him to a warm room as soon as you can, because he may have become dangerously chilled after even a short period of immersion in cold water.

Clear any debris *from his mouth with your finger*

✚ **If he is conscious,** simply comfort and reassure him, and make sure he keeps warm.

SHOCK

A life-threatening state of collapse, when blood pressure falls dangerously low, shock is a reaction to any severe injury, especially one in which your child has been badly burned or suffered heavy bleeding.

What can I do?

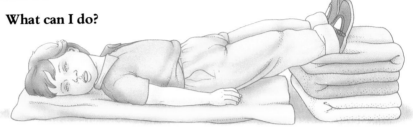

1 Lay your child down on her back, if possible on a coat or blanket. Turn her head to one side, then raise her feet about 20cm (8in) and rest them on something, such as a pile of clothes or a bag.
Don't raise her legs if she has a broken leg or a poisonous bite on her leg.

2 Cover her with a blanket or coat, or cuddle her, to keep her warm.
Don't try to warm her up with a hot water bottle or an electric blanket – this only draws blood away from the vital body organs to the skin.

3 If she complains of thirst, moisten her lips with a damp cloth.
Don't give her anything to eat or drink. There is one exception to this – you can give sips of water to your child if she has been badly burned.

4 If she becomes unconscious, check her breathing (see page 62).

✚ **If she is not breathing,** start artificial respiration (see pages 63–4).

✚ **If she is breathing,** put her into the recovery position (see page 65).

■ SYMPTOMS ■

▲ Pale, cold, sweaty skin
▲ blue or greyish tinge inside the lips or under the fingernails
▲ rapid and shallow breathing
▲ restlessness
▲ drowsiness or confusion
▲ unconsciousness.

■ EMERGENCY ■

Call for emergency help immediately if your child is in shock.

POISONING

Babies and young children tend to be curious and indiscriminating, so it is important to keep poisonous substances locked up and out of reach. Poisoning is one of the most common emergencies in young children.

What can I do?

1 If your child is unconscious, check his breathing (see page 62).

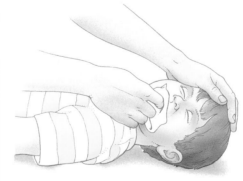

✚ **If he is not breathing,** start artificial respiration immediately (see pages 63–4), but wipe his face first (see above) or place a fine cloth over his mouth and breathe through that, to avoid getting any poison into your own mouth.

✚ **If he is breathing,** put him into the recovery position (see page 65).

■ EMERGENCY ■

Call for emergency help immediately if you think your child has swallowed something poisonous.

2 If you see signs of burning around your child's mouth, or have any other reason to think he may have swallowed a chemical product, wash his skin and lips with water. If he is conscious, give him some milk or water to drink.

3 Try to find out what he has taken, how much of it, and how long ago. Inform the doctor or ambulance staff and, if possible, give them a sample of the poison or its container.

4 If your child vomits, keep a small sample of the vomit and give it to the doctor or ambulance staff.
Don't try to make your child vomit.

■ SYMPTOMS ■

Your child's symptoms will depend on the type of poison he has swallowed. You may notice any of these signs:
▲ stomach pain
▲ vomiting
▲ symptoms of shock (see above)
▲ convulsions
▲ drowsiness
▲ unconsciousness
▲ burns or discoloration around the mouth if your child has swallowed a corrosive poison
▲ poison or empty container nearby.

BURNS AND SCALDS

A small, superficial burn, which causes reddening of the skin over an area of about 2 to 3cm (1in), is a minor burn, and can safely be treated at home. A burn that affects an area greater than this is a major burn, and is dangerous for your child, since fluid is lost from the damaged area, and infection can enter it. For sunburn, see page 53.

For sunburn, see page 53.

> ### EMERGENCY
> Get your child to hospital as soon as you have given first aid if:
> ▲ the burn covers an area of more than 2 to 3cm (about 1in)
> ▲ the burn was caused by an electric shock (see page 75).

MINOR BURNS
What can I do?

1 Cool the burn immediately, by holding it under cold, slowly running water until the pain decreases. This will help to prevent blisters developing.

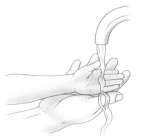

2 If a blister develops, put a pad of clean, non-fluffy material over it and hold it in place with sticking plaster or surgical tape.
Don't burst the blister – it protects the damaged area underneath while the new skin is growing.
Don't put any cream or lotion on the burn.

BURNING CLOTHES
What can I do?

1 Lay your child on the ground with the burning area uppermost. Avoid touching the burning area with your hands or your own clothes, if possible.

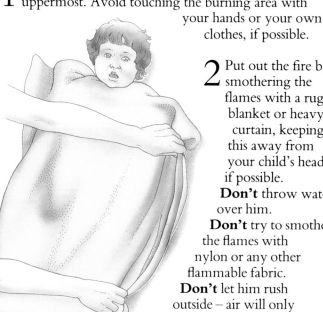

2 Put out the fire by smothering the flames with a rug, blanket or heavy curtain, keeping this away from your child's head if possible.
Don't throw water over him.
Don't try to smother the flames with nylon or any other flammable fabric.
Don't let him rush outside – air will only fan the flames.

3 When the flames are out, treat your child for a major burn (see right).

MAJOR BURNS
What can I do?

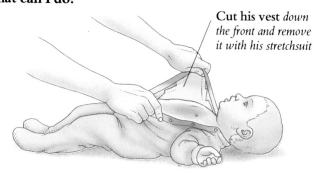

Cut his vest *down the front and remove it with his stretchsuit*

1 Remove any loose clothing which has been soaked in boiling water, fat or corrosive chemicals, taking care not to let it touch your child's skin anywhere else. Cut his clothes off rather than pull them over his face.
Don't remove dry, burnt clothing, or any clothing which has stuck to the burn.

2 Cool the burn immediately by drenching it with cold water: put your child in a cold bath or soak a sheet or towel in cold water and cover the burn with this.
Don't rub his skin.

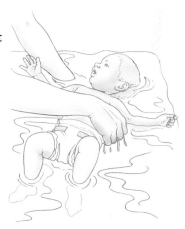

✚ **If chemicals have burnt his skin,** wash them off with plenty of cold water, but **don't** let the water run on to unharmed areas.

3 Cover the area very loosely with a clean, non-fluffy dressing. If you don't have a sterile dressing, an ironed handkerchief or pillow case will do.

4 Check for symptoms of shock, and treat your child for this if necessary (see opposite). If he complains of being thirsty, give him sips of water.

HEAVY BLEEDING

If blood spurts forcefully from a wound, or bleeding continues for more than five minutes, try to stem the flow so that the blood has a chance to clot.

What can I do?

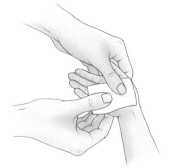
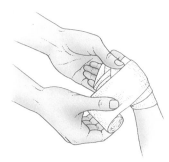

1 Raise the injured part above the level of your child's heart, to reduce the amount of blood flowing through it. Check for embedded objects in the wound; if there are any, treat them as described below.

2 Place a pad of clean, non-fluffy material over the wound – a clean handkerchief or teatowel is ideal, then press hard on it for about ten minutes. If there is no clean material available, press with your fingers, drawing the edges of the cut firmly together.

3 Leaving the original pad in place, bind a clean pad or dressing firmly over the wound so that the pressure is maintained. If this becomes soaked with blood, don't remove it, just bandage another pad over it, maintaining the pressure all the time.

> ■ **EMERGENCY** ■
>
> Get your child to hospital as soon as you have given first aid if he has been bleeding heavily.

4 Check for symptoms of shock (see page 68), and treat your child for this if necessary.

EMBEDDED OBJECTS

Small pieces of dirt in a cut will probably be washed out by bleeding, and larger pieces may wipe easily off the surface of the wound. However, if your child has something embedded in a wound, treat it as shown below.

What can I do?

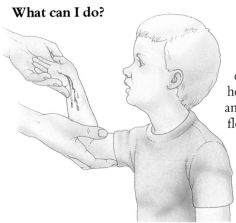

1 If your child's wound is bleeding heavily, raise the injured part above the level of his heart and apply pressure around the embedded object, not directly on it. If this seems to make the bleeding worse, release the pressure. **Don't** try to pull the object out and don't probe or try to clean the wound.

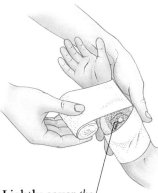

Lightly cover the embedded object and the fabric ring with a piece of gauze

> ■ **EMERGENCY** ■
>
> Take your child to hospital as soon as you have given first aid if he has something embedded in a wound.

2 Release the pressure for a moment, and roll up a small piece of material such as a clean handkerchief into a sausage shape, then twist this into a ring.

3 Place the ring of material round the cut and cover it with gauze, then bandage it in place firmly. **Don't** bandage tightly *over* the embedded object.

CUTS AND GRAZES

Cuts and grazes are common throughout childhood, and you can treat most of them yourself at home. Keep your child's tetanus injections up to date (see page 28), since tetanus can result from dirt entering a wound. Treat an animal bite as a cut, but if your child has a poisonous bite or sting, see page 76.

EMERGENCY

Take your child to hospital as soon as you have given first aid if:
▲ the cut is large or deep
▲ the cut has jagged or gaping edges
▲ your child has cut his face badly
▲ the cut or graze is very dirty
▲ your child has a puncture wound (a deep cut with only a small opening in the skin) caused by something dirty such as a rusty nail or an animal's tooth.
Consult your doctor as soon as possible if the area around the wound later becomes tender and red – it may be infected.

What can I do?

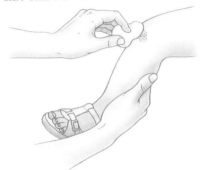 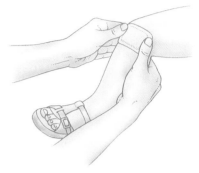

1 Wash your hands first, if possible. Clean the cut by holding it under running water, or wiping gently around it with an antiseptic wipe or cotton wool soaked in warm water. Use a clean piece of cotton wool for each stroke.
Don't remove anything that is embedded in the cut (see opposite).

✚ **If your child has been bitten by an animal,** wash the wound thoroughly with soap and water.

2 If the cut is still bleeding after five minutes, press a pad such as a clean handkerchief firmly on it for a few minutes.

3 Put a plaster or dressing over it, to help protect it and keep it clean.
Don't put any antiseptic ointment on your child's cut.

4 Keep the cut covered with sticking plaster or a dressing until it has completely healed. This ensures that the area remains moist, and helps the cut heal more quickly. Change the plaster or dressing every day – soak sticking plaster in water to remove it easily.

NOSE BLEEDS

Nose bleeds can result from a bump on the nose, nose-picking, or excessive nose-blowing. Sometimes there is no apparent reason for them. A few children seem prone to nose bleeds, probably because they have unusually fragile blood vessels in their noses.

CALL THE DOCTOR

Call your doctor now if your child's nose is still bleeding just as badly after half an hour. Consult your doctor if your child has frequent, severe nose bleeds.

What can I do?

1 Help your child to lean forwards over a bowl or wash-basin, and pinch her nostrils firmly together for about ten minutes. Try to stop her sniffing or swallowing the blood – encourage her to spit it out instead.

Pinch your child's nostrils firmly

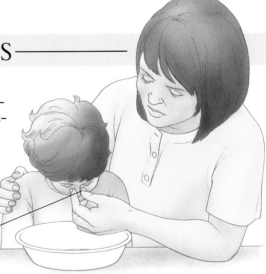

2 If her nose is still bleeding, hold a cloth wrung out in very cold water, or an ice pack wrapped in a cloth, over her nose for about two minutes, then pinch her nose again.

3 Don't blow your child's nose for about four hours after the bleeding has stopped.

HEAD AND FACE INJURY

Bumps on the head are common in young children, and may raise an impressive bruise, but are seldom serious. A cut on the forehead or scalp, even a very small one, is likely to bleed profusely.

If your child has had a severe blow to her head, she may suffer from concussion, which results when the brain is shaken within the skull, or from bleeding inside the skull – though this may not be apparent for several hours. Signs of these injuries are listed below.

EMERGENCY

Call for emergency help immediately if your child has injured her head and shows any unusual behaviour or has any of these symptoms up to 24 hours later:
- ▲ unconsciousness, however brief
- ▲ vomiting
- ▲ noisy breathing or snoring, if your child doesn't normally snore
- ▲ difficulty in waking, or abnormal drowsiness
- ▲ discharge of clear or blood-stained fluid from her nose or ear
- ▲ unusual crying
- ▲ severe headache
- ▲ dislike of bright light.

BROKEN TEETH

If your child has broken a tooth, or one has become dislodged, cover the tooth or broken piece with milk, and take your child and her tooth to your dentist or to hospital immediately.

What can I do?

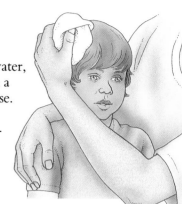

1 If your child's head is bruised, hold a cloth wrung out in very cold water, or an ice pack wrapped in a damp cloth, over the bruise. This may stop it swelling up. Check the skin underneath every minute, and remove the pack if a red patch with a white waxy centre develops.

2 If your child's head is bleeding, place a clean cloth over the cut and press on it, as for bleeding anywhere else on the body (see page 70).

3 Watch your child carefully for the next 24 hours, in case she develops any of the emergency signs listed in the box, left. If she bumped her head badly, wake her every three hours – if she won't wake up, **call for emergency help immediately**.

4 If a discharge of clear or blood-stained fluid trickles from your child's nose or ear, put her into the recovery position with a pad of clean material placed under her nose or ear. If the fluid is coming from her ear, lay her on the injured side, so that the fluid can drain away. **Don't** try to stop it trickling out.

BRUISES AND SWELLING

A bruise appears when a fall or blow causes bleeding into the tissues beneath the skin, which produces swelling and discoloration. Bruises normally fade gradually, and disappear after about a week.

CRUSHED FINGERS AND TOES

If your child has crushed his fingers in a door or window, or dropped something heavy on his foot, hold the injured area under cold running water for a few minutes. If it is very swollen, or is still painful after about half an hour, take your child to hospital.

What can I do?

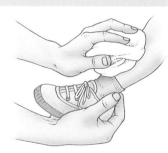

1 Hold a pad wrung out in very cold water, or an ice pack wrapped in a damp cloth, over the bruise for about half an hour. This should help to reduce pain and swelling.

2 If your child seems to be in great pain or if it hurts him to use a bruised limb, especially if the swelling is severe, check for any signs of a sprained joint or a broken bone (see opposite).

SPRAINED JOINTS

When a joint is sprained, the ligaments (tough fibres that support the joint) are damaged. This can cause symptoms very like those of a broken bone: if you are not sure which it is, treat as a broken bone (see below).

What can I do?

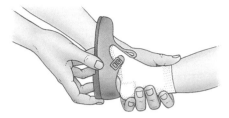

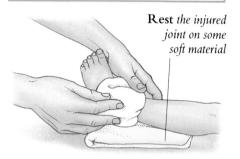

Rest the injured joint on some soft material

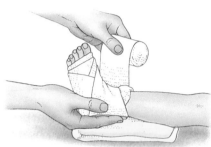

1 Gently take off your child's shoe and sock, or anything else that might constrict swelling around the injured joint.

2 Support the injured joint in the most comfortable position for your child, then hold a cloth wrung out in ice-cold water, or an ice pack wrapped in a damp cloth, on the joint, to reduce swelling and pain.

3 Wrap a thick layer of cotton wool round the joint, then bandage it firmly, but not so tightly that the beds of his toenails (or fingernails if you have bandaged his wrist or elbow) turn white or pale blue.

FRACTURES AND DISLOCATED JOINTS

Broken bones are unusual in babies and young children: their bones have not yet hardened, so they are flexible and tend to bend rather than break. Sometimes there may be a partial break, which mends easily (often called a "greenstick" fracture). A joint is dislocated if one or more bones have slipped out of place.

If you think your child's neck or back might be broken, do not move him or change his position unless he stops breathing (see pages 61–2).

What can I do?

1 Gently take off your child's shoe and sock, or anything else that might constrict swelling around the injured area.
Don't move him unless it is absolutely essential.

2 Support the injured part in the most comfortable position for your child.
For a broken wrist, arm or collar-bone, put padding round the injured area and, if your child will let you, gently fold his arm across his chest, then support it in a sling. Don't try to force his arm into this position.

Tie the bandages on the uninjured side

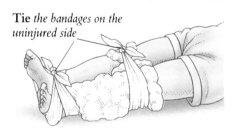

For a broken leg or ankle, lay your child down and put padding round the injured area and between his knees and ankles. Bandage the injured leg to the uninjured one, securing it above and below the injury. Put some padding under the knots.

3 Check for symptoms of shock and treat him for this if necessary (see page 68). If you think he has a broken leg, don't raise his legs.

FOREIGN BODY IN THE EYE

Eyelashes or particles of dust can easily get into the eye. If your child's eye seems irritated but you can't see anything in it, she may have an eye infection (see page 34).

SYMPTOMS

▲ Pain in the eye
▲ red, watering eye
▲ your child may rub her eye.

CHEMICALS IN THE EYE

If your child has splashed any chemicals or corrosive fluids in her eyes, wash her eyes out immediately under cold running water, keeping her eyelids apart with your fingers. If only one eye is affected, tilt her head so that the injured eye is lower, and the chemical cannot wash over into the uninjured one. Then cover the eye with a pad and take your child to hospital. If possible, take the chemical bottle with you.

What can I do?

1 Wait a few minutes to see if the natural watering of the eye washes the foreign body away. Try to stop your child rubbing her eye.

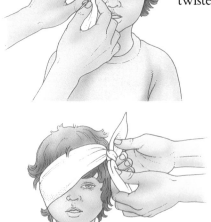

2 If the object is still there, examine your child's eye under a good light. Ask her to look up while you pull her lower eyelid gently down with your thumb.

3 If you can see the object on the white part of your child's eye, try to remove it by sweeping across it very gently with the corner of a clean handkerchief or a piece of damp, twisted cotton wool.

4 If you can see nothing, hold the eyelashes and draw the upper lid gently outwards and down over the lower lid. If the object is under the upper lid, this may dislodge it.

5 If your child's eye still feels gritty or painful, or if the object is not on the white of the eye, or not easily removable, cover the eye with a pad of cotton wool secured with a bandage or scarf and take her to hospital. Try to stop her rubbing her eye.
Don't try to remove anything on the central coloured part of the eye, or anything that is embedded in the white of the eye.

FOREIGN BODY IN THE EAR

Insects may crawl into your child's ear, and children sometimes push small objects into their ears. Don't let your child play with beads, marbles or similar small objects until he is old enough to understand that they should not be put into his ears.

SYMPTOMS

▲ Tickling in the ear
▲ partial deafness
▲ your child may rub or tug at his ear.

What can I do?

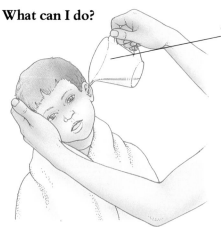

Tip the jug
very gently, so just a few drops go into his ear

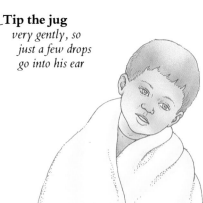

1 Put a towel round your child's shoulders, then hold his head on one side, with the affected ear on top, and pour a few drops of lukewarm water into his ear.

2 Tip his head the other way, so that the affected ear is underneath. The water may wash out whatever was in his ear. If this doesn't succeed, take your child to hospital.

FOREIGN BODY IN THE NOSE

Children sometimes stuff small pieces of food or other objects such as beads up their noses.

SYMPTOMS
▲ Smelly, blood-stained discharge from the nose.

What can I do?
If your child can blow his nose, help him to blow it, one nostril at a time. If this does not dislodge the object, don't try to remove it yourself – take your child to hospital straight away.

ELECTRIC SHOCK

A mild electric shock gives only a brief pins and needles sensation. A severe one can knock your child down, render her unconscious and stop both breathing and heartbeat. Electric current can also burn.

If your child touches a faulty appliance with wet hands, she will get a worse shock than touching it with dry hands.

EMERGENCY
Get your child to hospital as soon as you have given first aid if: ▲ she was unconscious, even if only for a few seconds   ▲ she has any electrical burns.

What can I do?

1 Switch off the current, at the mains if possible.

✚ **If you can't do this,** stand on an insulating material – such as a rubber mat or a pile of dry newspaper. Separate your child from the electrical source by pushing the cable or your child away, using some dry, non-conducting object such as a wooden chair or broom handle.

✚ **If nothing is available,** drag your child away, insulating your hand as much as you can by wrapping it in a dry cloth or newspaper. Grasp your child's clothes, and avoid touching her skin.

Move *the cable rather than your child's arm*

ELECTRICAL BURNS

Electricity can burn where the current enters the body and where it leaves, so your child may have burns where she touched the electrical source and anywhere that was in contact with the ground. Although these burns may look small, they are often very deep.

2 Check whether your child is conscious (see page 62).

✚ **If she is unconscious,** check her breathing: start artificial respiration immediately if necessary (see pages 63–4). If she is breathing, put her in the recovery position (see page 65).

✚ **If she is conscious,** comfort and reassure her. Check for symptoms of shock (see page 68).

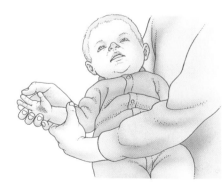

3 Examine her for any burns: check areas that were in contact with the electrical source or the ground (burns will look red or scorched, and may swell up). If you find any, treat them as major burns (see page 69).

MINOR BITES AND STINGS

Most plants, insects and jellyfish cause only minor stings which, while they may be painful, are not dangerous for your child. However, a few people develop a serious allergic reaction to stings, and therefore need urgent medical treatment.

SYMPTOMS
▲ Sharp pain
▲ redness
▲ slight swelling
▲ itching.

EMERGENCY
Get your child to hospital as soon as you have given first aid if he:
▲ has difficulty breathing
▲ develops a widespread rash with weals
▲ feels dizzy or faints
▲ develops symptoms of shock (see page 68)
▲ has a sting inside his mouth.

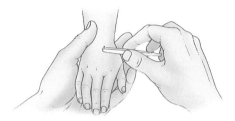

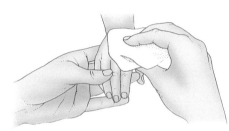

What can I do?

1 If your child has been stung by a bee, check whether the sting has been left in the skin. Scrape it off with a knife or fingernail, or pull it out with tweezers, taking care not to squeeze the tiny sac of poison.

2 Hold a cloth wrung out in ice-cold water over the sting.

✚ **If he has been stung in his mouth,** give him a cold drink or, if he is over two, let him suck an ice cube. This helps to reduce swelling.

3 Soothe the area around the sting, which will quickly become red, swollen and itchy, by dabbing it gently with cotton wool dipped in calamine lotion or surgical spirit, or by applying a little antihistamine ointment around the sting.

SNAKE AND SPIDER BITES, SCORPION STINGS

Snake bites, scorpion stings and the bites of poisonous spiders are always serious for young children.

Our most poisonous snakes are the cobra, the mamba, the berg-adder and the puff-adder. Parabuthus scorpions, with their thick tail sections and small pincers, are the most venomous.

SYMPTOMS
Your child's symptoms will de-pend on what has bitten or stung him; some symptoms may not appear for a few hours:
▲ severe pain
▲ one or two puncture marks
▲ swelling
▲ nausea or vomiting
▲ difficulty breathing
▲ shock (see page 68)
▲ convulsions
▲ drowsiness
▲ unconsciousness.

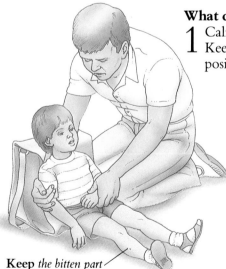

Keep the bitten part lower than his heart

EMERGENCY
Get your child to hospital as soon as you have given first aid if he has been bitten by a snake or spider, or stung by a scorpion.

What can I do?

1 Calm your child, and help him to sit down. Keep the bitten or stung part still, and position it below the level of his heart.

2 Wash thoroughly around the area, but **don't** suck the bite or sting.

3 Check for shock, and treat your child for this if necessary (see page 68). If he was bitten or stung on his leg or foot, don't raise his legs.

4 If he becomes unconscious, check his breathing (see page 62).

✚ **If he is not breathing,** start arti-ficial respiration (see pages 63–4).

✚ **If he is breathing,** put him into the recovery position (see page 65).

5 Try to identify the snake, spider or scorpion. If it has been caught, keep it to show to the doctor.

SEVERE JELLYFISH STINGS

The only jellyfish that gives a severe sting is the Portuguese man-of-war. It looks like a pale blue translucent sac floating in the water. If your child has been stung by one she will need medical attention.

What can I do?

1 If your child still has any of the stinging tentacles stuck to her skin, scrape them off using a handful of wet sand. Avoid touching the tentacles yourself.

2 Put your child into the recovery position (see page 65) and cover her with something dry.

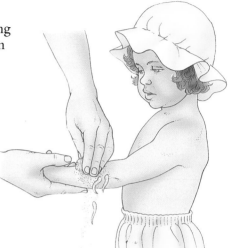

■ SYMPTOMS ■

▲ Burning pain
▲ redness
▲ shortness of breath
▲ fainting.

■ EMERGENCY ■

Get your child to hospital as soon as you have given first aid if she has a severe jellyfish sting.

THORNS AND SPLINTERS

Thorns or tiny splinters will frequently become embedded in your child's hands or feet. Those on his feet may not hurt, but splinters in the tips of his fingers will.

■ CALL THE DOCTOR ■

Consult your doctor as soon as possible if:
▲ the area around a splinter becomes red, swollen or tender up to 48 hours later
▲ you cannot remove a large or painful splinter
▲ your child has a splinter of glass or metal.

What can I do?

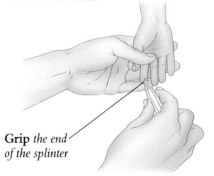

Grip *the end of the splinter*

1 If the end of the splinter is sticking out, sterilize a pair of tweezers in a flame, then pull the splinter straight out gently. Wash the area thoroughly with soap and water.

2 If there is no loose end, but you can see the splinter clearly, it is probably lying just below the surface of the skin. Sterilize a needle in a flame and let it cool, but don't touch the point. Then, starting where the splinter entered, gently tear the skin a little way along the line of the splinter. Carefully lift up the end of the splinter with the needle point and pull it out with tweezers, then wash the area thoroughly with soap and water.

3 If a small thorn or splinter has gone straight down into the skin, and is not painful, it is best to leave it alone. It will probably work its own way out in time.

BLISTERS

Blisters form when burns, scalds or friction damage the skin. The fluid-filled blister protects the new skin forming underneath. It will peel off of its own accord in a few days.

What can I do?

1 Don't burst or prick the blister. Dress your child in clothes that will not rub against it.

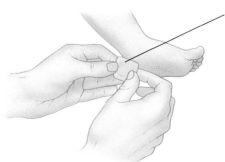

Cover the blister *with sticking plaster to prevent your child's shoe rubbing it*

2 If the blister bursts, leave it uncovered, unless it is likely to be exposed to further friction (for example, if it is on your child's foot). In this case, protect the blister with sticking plaster.

INDEX

A

abdomen: examination, 16, 44
  abdominal pain, 44
absence attacks, 57
accidents: first aid, 61–77
  life-saving techniques, 62–5
  safety precautions, 58–60
allergies: asthma, 42–3
  eczema, 52
  hives, 51
  nappy rash, 8
  stings, 76
ambulances, 61
anaesthetics, children, 17
animal bites, 71
ankles, injuries, 73
antibiotics, 21, 28
antibodies: and immunization, 28
  in newborn babies, 6
anxiety, and stomach pain, 44
appendicitis, 44
appetite: loss of, 6, 12
  sick children, 24
arms, fractures, 73
artificial respiration, 61, 62–4
aspirin, 22, 29
asthma, 42–3
  and eczema, 52
  and frequent chest infections, 40
attention lapses, 12

B

back injuries, 61
bacteria, in formula milk, 47
  see also gastro-enteritis
bacterial infections, 21
balanitis, 49
bandages, 61
barrier creams: and runny nose, 27
  and spots, 50
bathrooms, safety, 59
BCG immunization, 28
beakers, 24
bed rest, sick children, 25
bedrooms, safety in, 59
bee stings, 76
bites, 71, 76
bladder, infections, 48
bleeding: emergencies, 70
  nose bleeds, 71
blepharitis, 34
blisters, 77
  burns and scalds, 69
  cold sores, 54
blood, in stools, 45
boils, 50
bones, fractures, 73
bottle-feeding, adding sugar, 45
bottoms: genital problems, 49
  sore, 8
  see also nappy rash
bowels, normal movements in
  children, 45
  see also constipation; diarrhoea
brain: concussion, 72
  epilepsy, 57
  meningitis, 57

bread, for children, 45
breathing, 40
  artificial respiration, 62–3
  checking, 62
  emergencies, 6
  wheeziness, 40, 42
breathlessness, *see* asthma; bronchitis
broken bones, 73
bronchitis, 42
  and flu, 27
bruises, 72
brushes, hair, treating lice and nits, 56
burns, 69
  electrical, 75

C

cars, safety, 60
cat nets, 60
changing mat, 59
chapped skin, 53
chemicals: burns, 69
  in eyes, 74
chest: antibiotics to clear infections, 21
  external compression, 64
  flu and infections, 27
  infections, 27, 40–3
chicken pox, 31
  and antibiotics, 21
chilling, 10
choking, 66
circulation, checking, 64
circumcision, 49
clothes: baby, 10
  burning, 69
coeliac disease, 47
cold sores, 54
colds, 26–7
  and antibiotics, 21
colic, 6
collar-bones, fractures, 73
combs, treating lice and nits, 56
concussion, 72
conjunctivitis, 9, 34
constipation, in children, 45
convulsions: epilepsy, 57
  feverish, 20
  and immunization, 28
cot: death, 10
  safety, 59
cough, 40, 41
  whooping cough, 28, 33
cough medicines, 33, 41
cradle cap, 9
cradle, bouncing, 59
croup, 40
crushed fingers and toes, 72
crying, emergency sign, 6
cuts and grazes, 71

D

deafness, partial, 36–7
decongestants, 26
dehydration, 46
  in babies, 11
  in children, 24, 46–7
delirium, 20

diagnosing illness, 6–7, 12–13, 14–16
diarrhoea: in babies, 11
  in children, 47
  gastro-enteritis, 46–7
diet: for children, 45
  fibre, 45
digital thermometers 18–19
diphtheria, immunization, 28
discharges, vaginal, in babies and
  children, 49
dislocated joints, 73
doctors: examining children, 16
  when to call, 6, 14
drinks: and bottle-fed babies, 11
  encouraging sick child, 24
  to prevent dehydration, 11, 46, 47
droppers, medicine, 21
drops: ear, 23, 36
  eye, 23
  nose, 22, 26
drowning, 67
drugs and medicines:
  for children, 21–3
  drops, 22–3
  giving to babies, 21
  giving to children, 22

E

ears, 36
  drops, 23, 36
  foreign bodies, 74
  glue ear, 37
  middle ear infections, 37
  outer ear infections, 36
  wax in, 36
eczema, 52
  and ear infections, 36
electric shocks, 75
electrical burns, 75
electricity, safety, 60
embedded objects, 70
emergencies, accidents, 61–77
emergency signs: babies, 6
  children, 14
encephalitis, 57
entertaining sick children, 25
epilepsy, 57
  and immunization, 28
equipment: for children in
  hospital, 17
  for first aid, 61
external chest compression, 64
eyes: blepharitis, 34
  conjunctivitis, 34
  drops, 9, 23
  foreign bodies in, 74
  and measles, 30
  ointment, 23
  squints, 35
  sticky eye, 9
  styes, 35
  watering, 7

F

face injuries, 72
faeces, *see* stools
feeding: bottle-feeding, 11
  after gastro-enteritis, 11, 46
  sick children, 24
feet, plantar warts, 54–5
fever, 18–20
  aspirin and, 22, 29
  convulsions, 20
  delirium, 20
  reading a thermometer, 18
  reducing, 20
  signs of, 12
  taking temperature, 16, 19
fibre, 45
fingers, crushed, 72
first aid kit, 61
first aid techniques, 61–77
fits, *see* convulsions
flu, 26, 27
fontanelle: bulging, 57
  as emergency sign, 6, 57
  sunken, 6, 46
food, *see* diet
forceful vomiting, 11
foreign bodies: in ear, 74
  embedded in wounds, 70
  in eye, 74
  in nose, 75
foreskin, inflamed, 49
fractures, 73
fruit, and constipation, 45

G

garden, safety in, 60
gastro-enteritis, 25, 44, 46–7,
  in babies, 11
  bottle-feeding hygiene, 11, 47
  prevention, 11, 47
gates: garden, 60
  stair, 60
genitals, problems, 49
German measles (rubella), 29
  immunization, 28
  during pregnancy, 29
glands, swollen, 12
  feeling for, 15, 16
glue ear, 37
gluten, 47
grazes, 71
greenstick fractures, 73
grommets, 37

H

hair, lice and nits in, 56
hairbrushes, treating lice and nits, 56
halls, safety in, 60
hallucinations, 20
hands, and chilling, 10
hats: to prevent chilling, 10
  treating lice and nits, 56
hayfever, 12, 52

head: cradle cap, 9
  injuries, 72
  lice, 56
hearing, 36
  partial deafness, 36–7
heart: checking for beat, 64
  resuscitation, 62, 64
heat rash, 51
hernia, 7, 49
hiccups, 7
hives, 51
home, safety in, 58–60
hospitals: children in, 17
  emergencies, 61
hunger: see appetite
hygiene: bottle-feeding, 47
  and diarrhoea, 47
  and gastro-enteritis, 46–7
  solid food, 47

I

ice cubes, 24
ice lollies, ice, 24
illness: caring for a sick child, 24–5
  diagnosing, 6–7, 12–15
immunity: and breast-feeding, 6
  to infections, 6, 29
immunization, 28
  against flu, 27
impetigo, 55
infectious illnesss 29–33
  immunization, 28
  in young babies, 6
influenza, 26, 27
insect nets, 60
insect stings, 76
insects, in ears, 74
itchiness: and chicken pox, 31
  in children, 50

J

jellyfish stings, 77
joints: dislocated, 73
  sprained, 73

K

kidneys, 48
  infections, 48
kitchens, safety in, 58

L

lactose intolerance, 47
laxatives, 45
legs, fractures, 73
lice, 56
life-saving techniques, 62–5
lips, chapped, 53
living rooms, safety in, 60
lollies, 24
lungs, 42

lungs continued
  asthma, 42–3
  bronchitis, 42
  pneumonia, 43
  see also cough

M

major seizure, 57
measles, 30
  and antibodies, 21
  and colds, 26
  immunization, 28
medicines, see drugs
meningitis, 57
mercury thermometers, 18–19
milia, 7
milk spots, 7
moisturizers, 6
mouth: infections, 8, 38
  stings in, 76
mumps, 32
  and antibodies, 21
  immunization, 28

N

nappies, changing, 8, 59
nappy rash, 7, 8
  coping with, 8, 49
  and infection, 8, 49
navel, 7
nets, cat/insect, 60
nettle stings, 51
nits, 56
noses: drops, 22, 26
  foreign bodies in, 75
  nose bleeds, 71
  wiping, 26
nursing sick children, 24–5
nutrition, see diet

O

ointment, eye, 23
operations, children, 17
overheating, 10

P

pain: babies and children, 15
  as emergency sign, 6, 14
painkillers, 15
  aspirin, 22, 29
  paracetamol 20, 22, 29
pants: and genital infections, 49
  plastic, 8, 49
paracetamol, elixir, 20, 22, 29
penis, problems, 49
pertussis, see whooping cough
plantar warts, 54–5
plastic pants, 8, 49
play, sick children, 25
playpens, 58

pneumonia, 43
  and flu, 27
poisoning, 68
polio immunization, 28
premature babies: chilling, 10
  health care, 6
projectile vomiting, see forceful
  vomiting
pulse, 16, 64
pus, sticky eye, 9
pyloric stenosis, 11

R

rashes, 7, 8, 13, 15
  chicken pox, 31
  as emergency sign, 14
  German measles, 29
  heat rash, 51
  hives, 51
  impetigo, 55
  measles, 30
  nappy, 7, 8, 49
  newborn baby, 8
recovery position, 65
rest, see sleep
resuscitation, 61, 62–4
Reye's syndrome, 22, 29
rubella, see German measles

S

safety, 58–60
  in cars, 60
  in the garden, 60
  medicines, 22
  stairs, 60
salts, in glucose drink, 46
sandpits, 60
scalds, 69
scorpion stings, 76
scratching, 50
  and chicken pox, 31
seizures, see convulsions
shock, 61, 68
shocks, electric, 75
sickness, see vomiting
sinusitis, 26
skin: blisters, 77
  bruises, 72
  burns and scalds, 69
  chapped, 53
  chilling, 10
  cold sores, 54
  cuts and grazes, 71
  diagnosing problems, 50
  dry, 6
  eczema, 52
  heat rash, 51
  hives, 51
  impetigo, 55
  milk spots, 7
  overheating, 10
  spots and boils, 50
  sunburn, 53
  thorns and splinters, 77
  warts and plantar warts, 54–5
  see also itching; rashes

sleep, sick children, 25
slings, for fractures, 73
smoking: and asthma, 43
  and chest infections, 40
snake bites, 76
sore throats, 39
spider bites, 76
spinal injuries, 61
splinters, 77
sponging, tepid, 20
spoons, medicine, 21
spots, 50
  milk spots, 7
  newborn babies, 8
  see also rashes
sprained joints, 73
squints, 35
stairs: gates, 60
  safety, 60
sterilizing, bottle-feeding
  equipment, 46–7
stethoscope, 16
sticky eye, 9
stings, 76–7
stitches, in children, 17
stomach: pain, 44
  upsets, 11, 46–7
stools: abnormal, 44, 47
  blood in, 45
  emergency sign, 6
straws, drinking, 24
  and mumps, 32
  and sore mouth, 38
stye, 35
suffocation, 67
sugar, adding to bottle-feeds, 45
sun hats, 53
sunburn, 10, 53
surgery, and children, 17
sweating: babies, 10
  fevers, 20
  heat rash, 51
  overheating, 10
swellings, first aid, 72
swollen glands, 15, 16
symptoms, 6–7, 12–13, 14–16

T

tear ducts, blocked, 7
teeth, broken, 72
teething, and illness, 14
temperature: baby's room, 10
  bath water, 59
  chilling, 10
  emergencies, 6
  fever, 12, 16, 18–20, 29
  overheating, 10
  reducing a fever, 20
  taking a child's, 15, 18–19
temperature indicator strip, 18–19
tepid sponging, 20
testicles, 48
tetanus, 71, 76
  immunization, 28
thermometers, 18–19
thorns, 77
threadworms, 49, 56
throat infections, 39
  checking for, 15, 16

throat infections continued
  tonsillitis, 39
thrush, 8, 38, 49
toes, crushed, 72
tonsillitis, 39
toys, for sick children, 25
tuberculosis, immunization, 28
tummy ache, 44

U

unconsciousness, 61, 62–5
urinary system, 48
urinary system infections, 48
  and antibiotics, 21
  and stomach pain, 44

urination: frequent, 48
  painful, 48
urine, odd-coloured, 48
urticaria, 8, 51

V

vaccination, *see* immunization
vagina: discharges, 49
  problems in babies and children, 49
vegetables, fibre, 45
verrucas, *see* warts
virus diseases: and antibiotics, 21
  developing resistance, 26
  see also infectious illnesses

vomiting, 46
  babies, 11
  emergency sign, 6
  sick children, 24, 25

W

warts, 54–5
washing, nappies, 8
water: bath, 59
  safety, 60
watering eye, 7
wax in ears, 36
weight, baby's/child's, slow weight gain, 6
wheeziness, 40, 42

whooping cough, 33
  immunization, 28
windpipe, choking, 66
worms, threadworms, 49, 56
wounds: cuts and grazes, 71
  embedded objects, 70
  heavy bleeding, 70
wrists, fractures, 73

Z

zinc and castor oil cream, 27

ACKNOWLEDGMENTS

Picture credits
The publishers would like to thank the following for their kind permission to reproduce photographs:
(numbers indicate pages; t = top, b = below, c = centre, l = left, r = right)
Sue Ford, Western Opthalmic Hospital: 7tr, 9bl, 34r; National Medical Slide Bank: 7br, 30l, 34tl, 38bl, 50l, 51cl, 56l; St John's Institute of Dermatology: 52tl, 55tr; St Mary's Hospital: 9tl, 31tl and bl; Dr I. Williams: 6br, 7cr, 8t and cr, 29r, 35l, 39b, 51bl, 53br, 54t, bc and b.

Special photography
(numbers indicate pages; t = top, b = below, c = centre, l = left, r = right)
Dave King: 1, 4: 1st column pictures 2–4, 2nd column pictures 1–4, 5, 6t and l 8b, 9tr, cr and br, 10–28, 29r, 30t, cr and b, 31tr and br, 32–3, 34br, 35tr and b, 36–7, 38tl, tr and cr, 39t, 41–9, 50c and r, 51t and bl, 52cl, cr and b, 53tl, tr and bl, 54tl and cr, 55tl, cr and b, 56c and r, 58t, 61;
Ray Moller: 7c
Stephen Oliver: 4: 1st column pictures 1 and 5;
Steve Shott: 4: 2nd column picture 5.

Location photography
Staff of AMI Portland Hospital: Claire Jackaman, Vivien Gibbs, Cheryl Leach and new mothers; staff of Kingston General Hospital: Elizabeth Cole, Miss Moyle, Linda Hodges, Miss Farrington.

Make-up
Nicky Freeman; Bettina Graham; Barbara Jones; Ellen Kramer; Mary-Lou; Sue Sian.

Loan or supply of props
Boots Baby Business Centre; Children's World; Ohmeda; Pan Servico Surgical; Porter Nash; Seward Medical; Jacob White Hospital Equipment.

Illustrators
Coral Mula: all line artwork except pp 58–60; Jim Robins: 58–60.

Airbrushing
Trevor Hill; also Roy Flooks, Brian Sayers and Graham Smith.

Editorial help
Ruth Carim; Pauline Frost; Clare Mitchison; Dr Frances Williams.

Design help
Hannah Moore; Margaret Sadler; Michelle Walker.

Picture research
Derek, Clive and Neil Bromhall at Genesis Film Productions Ltd; Marian Hudson, Medical Illustration Department, Charing Cross Hospital; Sandra Schneider; Tim Woodcock.

Index
Hilary Byrd.